I0781571

Welcome to the ***"Mind Diet Cookbook for Seniors Over 60: 115+ Nutrient-Packed Recipes to Support Mental Acuity and Brain Health."*** *This cookbook is a comprehensive guide designed specifically for older adults who are looking to enhance cognitive function, support brain health, and promote overall well-being through nutrition.*

As we age, maintaining mental acuity becomes increasingly important. The Mind Diet, which stands for Mediterranean-DASH Intervention for Neurodegenerative Delay, emphasizes foods that are known to be beneficial for brain health. This includes a focus on fruits, vegetables, whole grains, lean proteins, and healthy fats, all of which are rich in vitamins, minerals, and antioxidants that support cognitive function.

The recipes in this cookbook are crafted with these principles in mind. Each dish is not only delicious but also designed to incorporate ingredients that are known to benefit brain health. From vibrant salads and hearty soups to satisfying main courses and nutritious snacks, you'll find a variety of recipes that make it easy to follow the Mind Diet and enjoy meals that support your cognitive wellness.

Whether you're new to the Mind Diet or looking to expand your repertoire of brain-boosting recipes, this cookbook offers a wealth of options to suit every taste and occasion. Our goal is to empower you to take control of your brain health through the food you eat, making it both enjoyable and beneficial to support your mental clarity and vitality.

Join us on a journey to nourish your brain, enhance your cognitive function, and embrace a lifestyle that promotes healthy aging. Let the Mind Diet Cookbook be your guide to delicious and nutritious meals that support your well-being well into your golden years. Here's to eating well and living well!

Warm regards,

Eating well is crucial for maintaining health and vitality as we age, especially for individuals over 60. Here are some important notes to keep in mind when eating for elderly adults:

1. Nutrient Density: Choose foods that are nutrient-dense, meaning they provide a high amount of vitamins, minerals, and other essential nutrients relative to their calorie content. This helps ensure that every bite counts towards meeting nutritional needs.

2. Balanced Diet: Aim for a balanced diet that includes a variety of food groups:
- Fruits and Vegetables: Rich in vitamins, minerals, and antioxidants.
- Whole Grains: Provide fiber for digestive health and sustained energy.
- Lean Proteins: Sources like fish, poultry, beans, and legumes for muscle strength and repair.
- Healthy Fats: Found in olive oil, nuts, seeds, and fatty fish like salmon, supporting heart health and cognitive function.

3. Hydration: Encourage adequate fluid intake, as older adults may have a decreased sense of thirst. Water, herbal teas, and broths can help maintain hydration levels.

4. Portion Control: Adjust portion sizes to meet individual energy needs, which may decrease with age due to changes in metabolism and activity levels.

5. Fiber and Digestive Health: Include fiber-rich foods like whole grains, fruits, and vegetables to support digestive health and prevent constipation, a common issue among seniors.

6. Calcium and Vitamin D: Ensure adequate intake of calcium and vitamin D for bone health. Sources include dairy products, fortified foods, and sunlight exposure for vitamin D synthesis.

7. Mindful Eating: Practice mindful eating to savor food, aid digestion, and recognize satiety cues, which can help prevent overeating.

8. Limit Sodium and Sugar: Reduce intake of processed foods high in sodium and added sugars, which can contribute to hypertension, diabetes, and other health issues.

9. Regular Meals: Encourage regular meals and snacks to maintain energy levels throughout the day. Aim for consistency in meal times to support digestive health.

10. Consultation with Healthcare Provider: Individual dietary needs may vary based on health conditions, medications, and personal preferences. Regular consultations with a healthcare provider or registered dietitian can provide personalized guidance and support.

By following these notes and maintaining a well-balanced diet, elderly individuals can support their overall health, energy levels, and quality of life as they age gracefully.

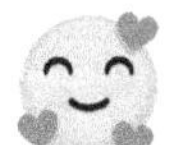 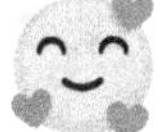 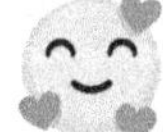 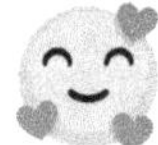 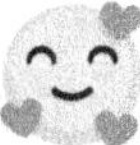 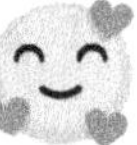 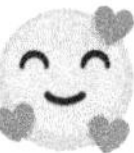 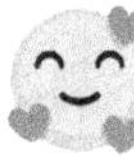  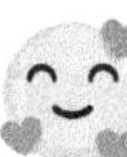

1. Greek yogurt with berries and nuts

Let's do that and fill in the time here   Prep Time :   Cook Time :   Servings :

Is this dish easy or difficult for you to make?

 ◯   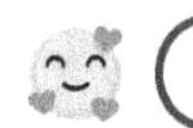 ◯

Write 5 ....
friends
with   ....
whom
you   ....
want to
share   ....
this
dish   ....

INGREDIENTS

- 1 cup plain Greek yogurt
- 1/2 cup mixed berries (such as blueberries, raspberries, and/or blackberries)
- 2 tablespoons chopped walnuts or almonds

1. Spoon the Greek yogurt into a bowl.

2. Top the yogurt with the mixed berries.

3. Sprinkle the chopped nuts over the top.

This dish provides the following benefits for seniors over 60 following the MIND diet:

- Greek yogurt is an excellent source of protein, which is important for maintaining muscle mass and strength as we age.

- Berries are rich in antioxidants and have been shown to have neuroprotective effects, which can help support brain health.

- Nuts, such as walnuts and almonds, are a good source of healthy fats, fiber, and various vitamins and minerals that are important for cognitive function.

The MIND diet emphasizes the consumption of foods that have been linked to a reduced risk of cognitive decline and Alzheimer's disease, including berries, nuts, and dairy products like Greek yogurt. This simple and delicious recipe checks all those boxes, making it a great option for seniors looking to support their brain health.

How would you rate this dish?

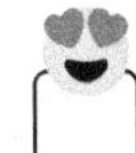 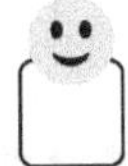 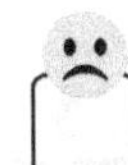 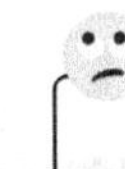 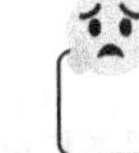

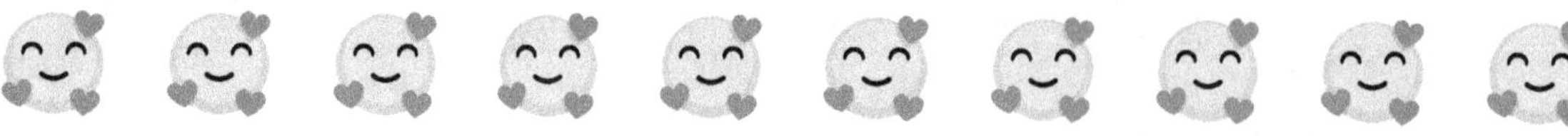

2. Oatmeal with sliced almonds and blueberries

Let's do that and fill in the time here — Prep Time : — Cook Time : — Servings :

Is this dish easy or difficult for you to make?

 ◯   ◯

Write 5 friends with whom you want to share this dish

....

....

....

....

....

INGREDIENTS

- 1 cup old-fashioned oats
- 1 1/2 cups unsweetened almond milk (or milk of your choice)
- 1/4 cup sliced almonds
- 1/2 cup fresh or frozen blueberries
- 1 teaspoon honey (optional)

1. In a medium saucepan, combine the oats and almond milk. Bring to a simmer over medium heat, stirring occasionally, until the oats are tender and the mixture has thickened, about 5-7 minutes.

2. Remove the oatmeal from the heat and stir in the sliced almonds and blueberries.

3. If desired, drizzle the honey over the top.

This dish provides the following benefits for seniors over 60 following the MIND diet:

- Oats are a whole grain that are rich in fiber, which can help support digestive health and feelings of fullness.

- Almonds are a good source of healthy fats, protein, and various vitamins and minerals that are important for brain health, such as vitamin E and magnesium.

- Blueberries are a powerful antioxidant and have been shown to have neuroprotective effects, which can help support cognitive function.

The MIND diet emphasizes the consumption of whole grains, nuts, and berries, all of which are included in this recipe. This simple and delicious breakfast option can be a great way for seniors to start their day with a brain-healthy meal.

How would you rate this dish?

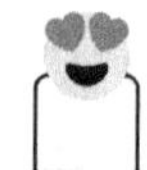 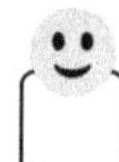  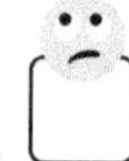 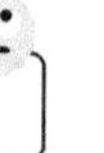 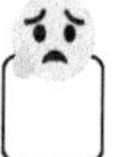

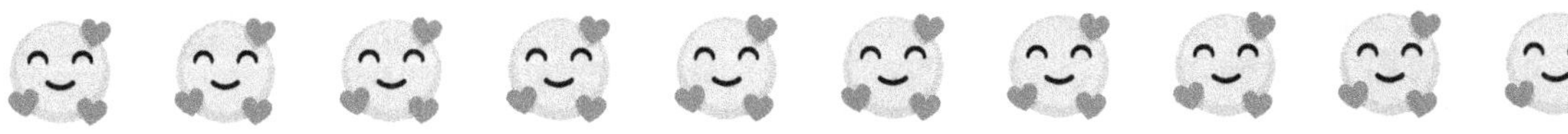

3. Whole-grain toast with avocado and tomato

 Prep Time :   Cook Time :   Servings :

Is this dish easy or difficult for you to make?

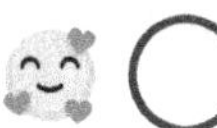 ○   ○

Write 5 friends with whom you want to share this dish
....
....
....
....
....

INGREDIENTS

- 2 slices of whole-grain bread, toasted
- 1/2 ripe avocado, mashed
- 1-2 sliced tomatoes
- Salt and pepper to taste

1. Toast the whole-grain bread until lightly golden brown.

2. Spread the mashed avocado evenly over the toasted bread slices.

3. Top the avocado with sliced tomatoes.

4. Season with a pinch of salt and freshly ground black pepper.

This makes for a nutritious and satisfying breakfast or snack. The whole grains provide fiber, the avocado offers healthy fats, and the tomatoes add vitamins and antioxidants. It's a simple but delicious way to enjoy some wholesome ingredients.

How would you rate this dish?

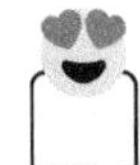 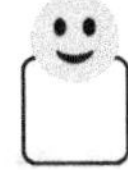 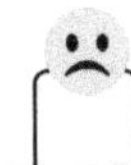 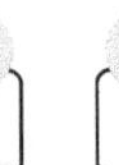 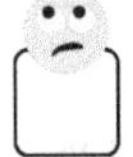 

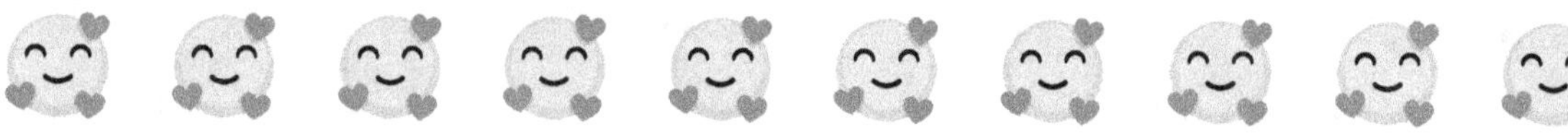

4. Scrambled eggs with spinach and feta

Let's do that and fill in the time here  Prep Time :   Cook Time :   Servings :

Is this dish easy or difficult for you to make?

 ◯   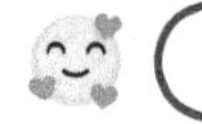 ◯

Write 5 friends with whom you want to share this dish

....

....

....

....

....

INGREDIENTS

- 6 large eggs
- 2 tbsp milk or unsweetened almond milk
- 1 tsp olive oil
- 2 cups fresh spinach, chopped
- 2 oz crumbled feta cheese
- Salt and pepper to taste

1. In a medium bowl, whisk together the eggs and milk until well combined.

2. Heat the olive oil in a nonstick skillet over medium heat.

3. Add the chopped spinach and sauté for 2-3 minutes until wilted.

4. Pour in the egg mixture and let it sit for 20-30 seconds to set the bottom.

5. Using a spatula, gently push the cooked egg towards the center, tilting the pan to allow the uncooked egg to flow to the edges.

6. Continue this process, gently folding and stirring the eggs, until they are softly scrambled and no longer runny, about 2-3 minutes total.

7. Remove from heat and stir in the crumbled feta. Season with salt and pepper to taste. Serve immediately.

This recipe supports the MIND diet for seniors in a few key ways:

- Eggs are a great source of protein, vitamins, and minerals important for brain health.

- Spinach is high in folate, vitamin K, and antioxidants that can help slow cognitive decline.

- Feta cheese provides beneficial probiotics and healthy fats.

- The MIND diet emphasizes plant-based foods like vegetables, fruits, whole grains, nuts, and olive oil.

How would you rate this dish?

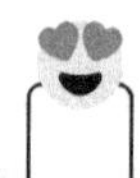 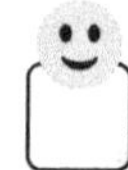 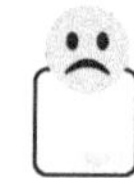 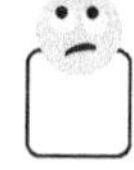 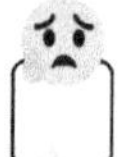

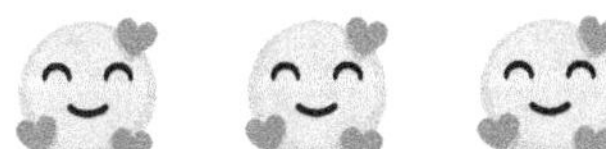

5. Smoothie with spinach, berries, and almond milk

Let's do that and fill in the time here  Prep Time :   Cook Time :   Servings :

Is this dish easy or difficult for you to make?

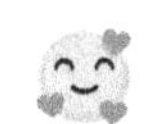 ◯   ◯

Write 5 friends with whom you want to share this dish

....

....

....

....

....

INGREDIENTS

- 1 cup fresh spinach leaves
- 1 cup frozen mixed berries (such as strawberries, blueberries, raspberries)
- 1 cup unsweetened almond milk
- 1 tablespoon honey or maple syrup (optional)
- 1/2 cup ice cubes

1. Add the spinach, frozen berries, almond milk, and honey/maple syrup (if using) to a high-powered blender.

2. Blend on high speed until the mixture is smooth and creamy, about 1-2 minutes.

3. Add the ice cubes and blend again until the smoothie is thick and frosty.

4. Pour into a glass and enjoy immediately.

Tips:

- You can use fresh or frozen berries. Frozen will make the smoothie thicker.

- Add a tablespoon of nut butter or a scoop of protein powder for extra nutrition.

- Adjust sweetener to taste, depending on the sweetness of your berries.

- For a creamier texture, use 1/2 cup almond milk and 1/2 cup plain Greek yogurt.

How would you rate this dish?

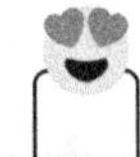 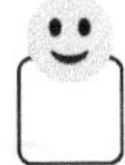  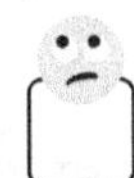 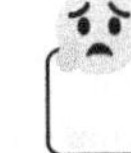

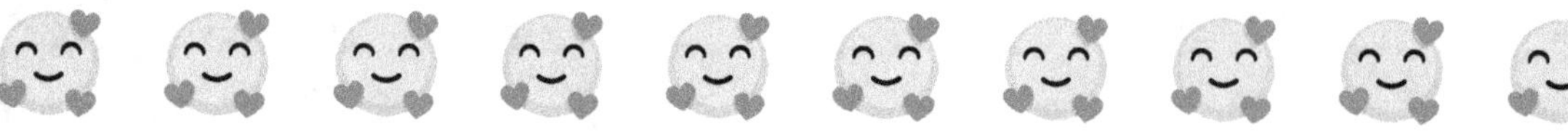

6. Whole-grain pancakes with fresh fruit

Prep Time :   Cook Time :   Servings :

Is this dish easy or difficult for you to make?

 ◯   ◯

Write 5 friends with whom you want to share this dish ....

INGREDIENTS

- 1 cup whole-wheat flour
- 1/2 cup rolled oats
- 1 teaspoon baking powder
- 1/2 teaspoon baking soda
- 1/4 teaspoon salt
- 1 egg
- 1 cup low-fat milk
- 1 tablespoon honey or maple syrup
- 1 teaspoon vanilla extract
- 2 cups mixed fresh berries (such as blueberries, raspberries, strawberries)

How would you rate this dish?

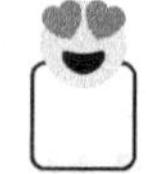 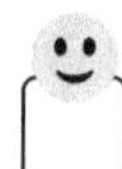 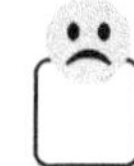 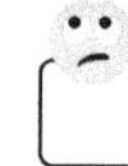 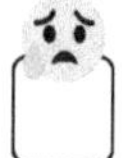

1. In a large bowl, whisk together the whole-wheat flour, rolled oats, baking powder, baking soda, and salt.

2. In a separate bowl, beat the egg. Then stir in the milk, honey/maple syrup, and vanilla.

3. Pour the wet ingredients into the dry ingredients and stir just until combined (do not overmix).

4. Heat a lightly oiled griddle or nonstick skillet over medium heat.

5. For each pancake, pour about 1/4 cup of the batter onto the griddle. Cook for 2-3 minutes per side, until golden brown.

6. Serve the pancakes warm, topped with the fresh mixed berries.

This recipe supports the MIND diet for seniors in the following ways:

- Whole grains (whole-wheat flour, rolled oats) provide complex carbs, fiber, and B vitamins.

- Berries are rich in antioxidants and may help protect brain health.

- Low-fat milk provides protein and calcium.

- Honey/maple syrup provide natural sweetness without refined sugar.

Enjoy this nutritious and delicious breakfast!

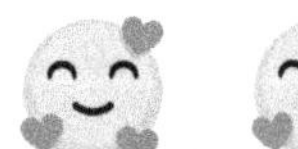 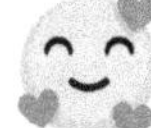 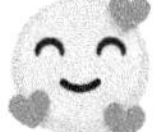 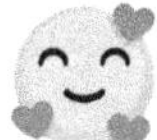 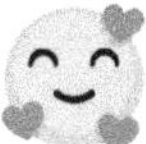 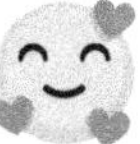 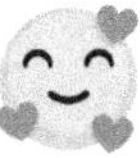 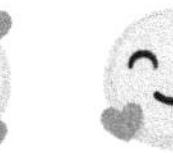 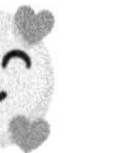 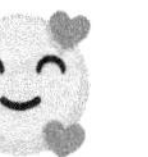 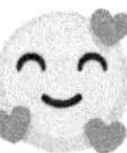

7. Chia seed pudding with almond milk and strawberries

Prep Time :   Cook Time :   Servings :

Is this dish easy or difficult for you to make?

Write 5 ....
friends
with ....
whom
you ....
want to
share ....
this
dish ....

INGREDIENTS

- 1/4 cup chia seeds
- 1 cup unsweetened almond milk
- 1 tablespoon honey or maple syrup (optional)
- 1 teaspoon vanilla extract
- 1 cup fresh strawberries, sliced

1. In a medium bowl, whisk together the chia seeds, almond milk, honey/maple syrup (if using), and vanilla extract until well combined.

2. Cover the bowl and refrigerate for at least 2 hours, or overnight, stirring occasionally, until the chia seeds have thickened the mixture into a pudding-like consistency.

3. When ready to serve, divide the chia seed pudding into 2-3 serving bowls or glasses.

4. Top each serving with sliced fresh strawberries.

5. Serve chilled.

Optional Variations:

- Use a different type of milk (dairy, coconut, etc.) instead of almond milk.

- Add a sprinkle of cinnamon or nutmeg on top.

- Mix in other fresh or frozen berries, such as blueberries or raspberries.

- Top with chopped nuts, shredded coconut, or a drizzle of nut butter.

This chia seed pudding is a nutritious and delicious breakfast or snack. The chia seeds provide fiber, protein, and omega-3 fatty acids, while the almond milk and strawberries offer additional vitamins, minerals, and antioxidants. It's a great option for a healthy, easy-to-prepare meal.

How would you rate this dish?

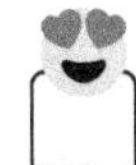 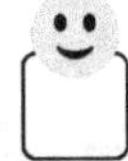 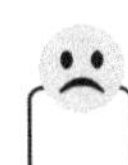 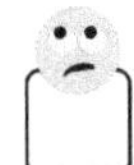 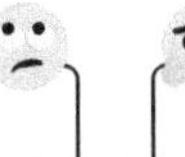

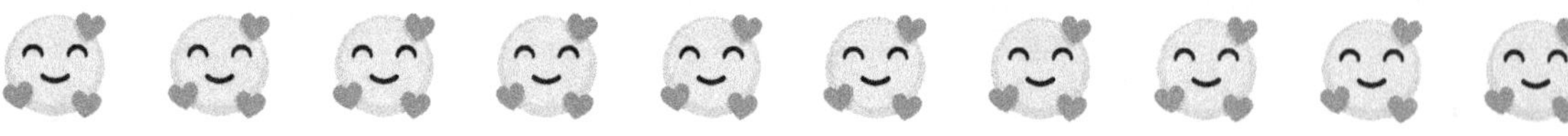

8. Quinoa breakfast bowl with walnuts and raspberries

Let's do that and fill in the time here  Prep Time :   Cook Time :   Servings :

Is this dish easy or difficult for you to make?

 ◯   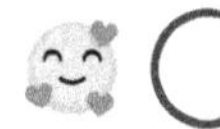 ◯

Write 5 friends with whom you want to share this dish

....

....

....

....

....

INGREDIENTS

- 1 cup cooked quinoa, cooled
- 1/2 cup unsweetened almond milk
- 1 tablespoon honey or maple syrup (optional)
- 1/4 cup fresh raspberries
- 2 tablespoons chopped walnuts
- 1 teaspoon ground cinnamon

1. In a medium bowl, combine the cooked quinoa, almond milk, and honey/maple syrup (if using). Stir to mix well.

2. Top the quinoa mixture with the fresh raspberries, chopped walnuts, and ground cinnamon.

3. Serve immediately, or refrigerate until ready to eat.

This quinoa breakfast bowl supports the MIND diet for seniors in the following ways:

- Quinoa is a whole grain that provides complex carbs, fiber, protein, and B vitamins.

- Walnuts are a good source of healthy fats, including omega-3s, which are important for brain health.

- Raspberries are rich in antioxidants and may help protect cognitive function.

- Almond milk is a dairy-free, low-fat option that provides calcium and vitamin E.

- Cinnamon is an anti-inflammatory spice that may also have cognitive benefits.

The combination of nutrient-dense ingredients in this recipe makes it an excellent breakfast choice for seniors following the MIND diet. It's easy to prepare, satisfying, and supports overall brain health.

How would you rate this dish?

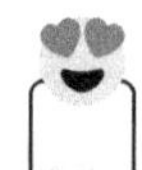 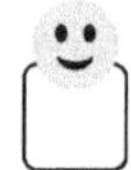 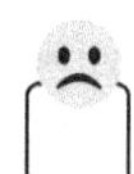 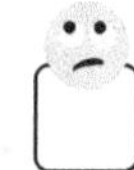 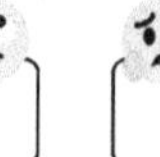

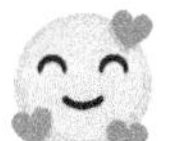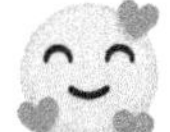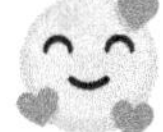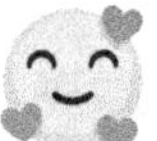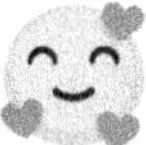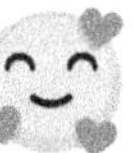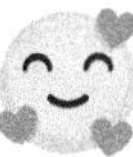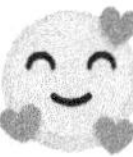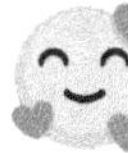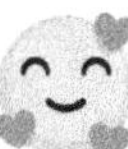

9. Cottage cheese with peaches and chia seeds

Let's do that and fill in the time here 🕐 Prep Time :   🕐 Cook Time :   🍴 Servings :

Is this dish easy or difficult for you to make?

 ◯   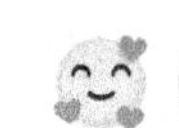 ◯

Write 5 friends with whom you want to share this dish

....

....

....

....

....

INGREDIENTS

- 1 cup low-fat cottage cheese
- 1 medium peach, sliced
- 1 tablespoon chia seeds
- 1 teaspoon honey or maple syrup (optional)
- Ground cinnamon (optional)

1. In a bowl, combine the cottage cheese and sliced peaches.

2. Sprinkle the chia seeds over the top.

3. Drizzle with honey or maple syrup, if desired.

4. Optionally, add a light dusting of ground cinnamon.

This cottage cheese dish supports the MIND diet for seniors in the following ways:

- Cottage cheese is a good source of protein, which is important for maintaining muscle mass and strength as we age.

- Peaches are a fruit rich in antioxidants, vitamins, and fiber, which can help support brain health.

- Chia seeds are high in omega-3 fatty acids, which are beneficial for cognitive function.

- Cinnamon is an anti-inflammatory spice that may also have positive effects on the brain.

The MIND diet emphasizes the consumption of whole, plant-based foods like fruits, vegetables, whole grains, nuts, and seeds. This cottage cheese dish checks all those boxes, making it a nutritious and delicious option for seniors looking to support their brain health.

You can adjust the sweetness by adding more or less honey/maple syrup, depending on your personal preference. This dish can be enjoyed as a healthy breakfast, snack, or even a light dessert.

How would you rate this dish?

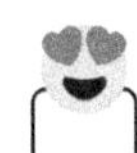 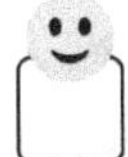  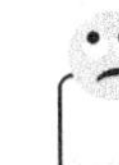 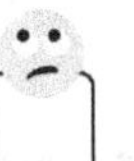 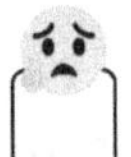

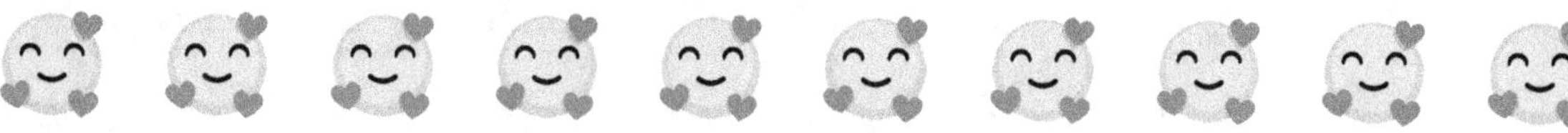

10. Spinach and mushroom omelet

Prep Time :   Cook Time :   Servings :

Is this dish easy or difficult for you to make?

 ◯   ◯

Write 5 ....
friends
with ....
whom
you ....
want to
share ....
this
dish ....

INGREDIENTS

- 3 eggs
- 1 tablespoon unsweetened almond milk (or low-fat milk)
- 1/4 teaspoon salt
- 1/4 teaspoon ground black pepper
- 1 cup fresh spinach leaves, chopped
- 1/2 cup sliced mushrooms
- 1 tablespoon grated Parmesan cheese (optional)

How would you rate this dish?

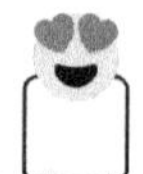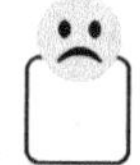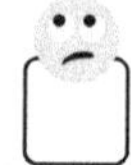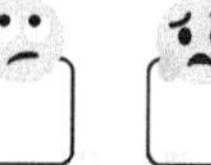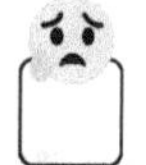

1. In a small bowl, whisk together the eggs, almond milk, salt, and pepper until well combined.

2. Heat a nonstick skillet over medium heat and spray with a small amount of cooking spray or olive oil.

3. Pour the egg mixture into the skillet and let it cook for 1-2 minutes, until the edges start to set.

4. Sprinkle the chopped spinach and sliced mushrooms over the top of the eggs.

5. Use a spatula to gently fold the omelet in half, then slide it onto a plate.Optionally, top the omelet with the grated Parmesan cheese.

This spinach and mushroom omelet supports the MIND diet for seniors in the following ways:

- Spinach is a leafy green vegetable that is rich in vitamins, minerals, and antioxidants, which are important for brain health.

- Mushrooms contain compounds that may help protect the brain and reduce inflammation.

- Eggs are a good source of protein, which is essential for maintaining muscle mass and strength.

- Parmesan cheese provides additional protein and calcium, which are both important nutrients for older adults.

The MIND diet emphasizes the consumption of whole, plant-based foods, and this omelet recipe checks all those boxes. It's a delicious and nutritious breakfast option that can help support cognitive function and overall health for seniors.

11. Quinoa salad with black beans, corn, and avocado

Let's do that and fill in the time here  Prep Time :   Cook Time :   Servings :

Is this dish easy or difficult for you to make?

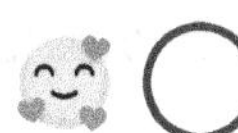

Write 5 friends with whom you want to share this dish
....
....
....
....
....

INGREDIENTS

- 1 cup cooked quinoa, cooled
- 1 (15 oz) can black beans, rinsed and drained
- 1 cup frozen corn kernels, thawed
- 1 avocado, diced
- 1/4 cup chopped fresh cilantro
- 2 tablespoons olive oil
- 2 tablespoons lime juice
- 1/2 teaspoon ground cumin
- 1/4 teaspoon salt
- 1/4 teaspoon black pepper

1. In a large bowl, combine the cooked quinoa, black beans, corn, avocado, and cilantro.

2. In a small bowl, whisk together the olive oil, lime juice, cumin, salt, and pepper.

3. Pour the dressing over the quinoa mixture and gently toss to coat everything evenly.

4. Serve chilled or at room temperature.

This quinoa salad supports the MIND diet for seniors in the following ways:

- Quinoa is a whole grain that provides complex carbs, fiber, and protein.

- Black beans are a good source of plant-based protein, fiber, and antioxidants.

- Corn is a vegetable that contains vitamins, minerals, and antioxidants.

- Avocado is a healthy fat that can help improve brain function and cognitive health.

- Cilantro is an herb that may have anti-inflammatory properties and support brain health.

The MIND diet emphasizes the consumption of whole, plant-based foods, and this quinoa salad checks all those boxes. It's a nutritious and delicious option that can be enjoyed as a main dish or a side salad.

How would you rate this dish?

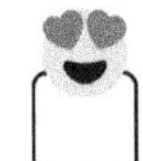 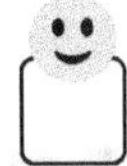 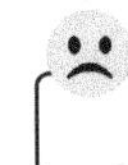 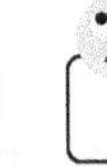 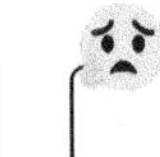

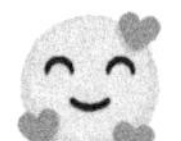 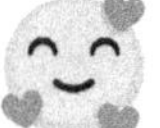 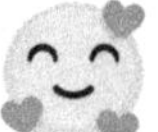 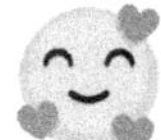 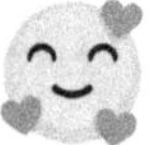 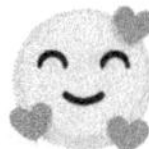 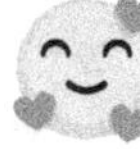 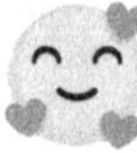 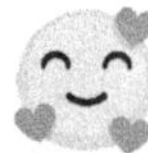 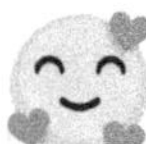

12. Lentil soup with vegetables

Let's do that and fill in the time here  Prep Time :   Cook Time :   Servings :

Is this dish easy or difficult for you to make?

 ◯   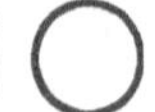 ◯

Write 5 friends with whom you want to share this dish

....

....

....

....

....

INGREDIENTS

- 1 tablespoon olive oil
- 1 onion, diced
- 3 cloves garlic, minced
- 2 carrots, peeled and diced
- 2 celery stalks, diced
- 1 cup green or brown lentils, rinsed
- 4 cups low-sodium vegetable or chicken broth
- 1 (14.5 oz) can diced tomatoes
- 2 cups chopped kale or spinach
- 1 teaspoon dried thyme
- 1/2 teaspoon dried rosemary
- Salt and black pepper to taste

1. In a large pot or Dutch oven, heat the olive oil over medium heat. Add the onion and sauté for 3-4 minutes until translucent.

2. Add the garlic, carrots, and celery. Sauté for an additional 2-3 minutes.

3. Stir in the lentils, broth, diced tomatoes, kale/spinach, thyme, and rosemary. Season with salt and pepper to taste.

4. Bring the soup to a boil, then reduce heat and simmer for 20-25 minutes, or until the lentils are tender.

5. Serve hot, garnished with additional chopped kale/spinach if desired.

This lentil soup supports the MIND diet for seniors in the following ways:

- Lentils are a legume that provide plant-based protein, fiber, and complex carbs.

- Vegetables like carrots, celery, onions, and leafy greens are rich in vitamins, minerals, and antioxidants.

- Herbs like thyme and rosemary have anti-inflammatory properties that may benefit brain health.

- The overall nutrient-dense composition of this soup aligns with the MIND diet's emphasis on whole, plant-based foods.

Lentil soup is a comforting, easy-to-prepare meal that can be enjoyed throughout the week. It's a great option for seniors looking to support their cognitive function and overall health.

How would you rate this dish?

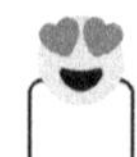    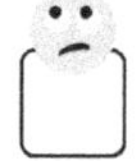 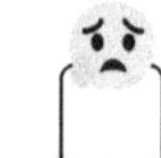

 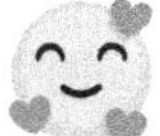  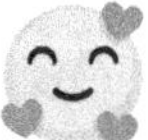 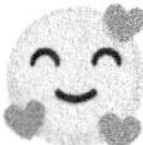 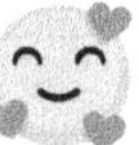 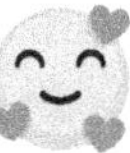 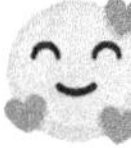 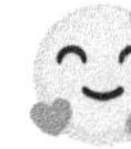 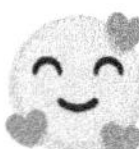

13. Greek salad with olive oil and lemon dressing

Let's do that and fill in the time here   Prep Time :   Cook Time :   Servings :

Is this dish easy or difficult for you to make?

 ◯   ◯

Write 5 friends with whom you want to share this dish

....
....
....
....

INGREDIENTS

Salad:
- 5 cups chopped romaine lettuce
- 1 cup cherry tomatoes, halved
- 1/2 cucumber, diced
- 1/2 red onion, thinly sliced
- 1/2 cup pitted kalamata olives, halved
- 1/2 cup crumbled feta cheese

Dressing:
- 3 tablespoons extra-virgin olive oil
- 2 tablespoons fresh lemon juice
- 1 teaspoon Dijon mustard
- 1 garlic clove, minced
- 1/4 teaspoon dried oregano
- Salt and black pepper to taste

1. In a large salad bowl, combine the chopped romaine, cherry tomatoes, cucumber, red onion, kalamata olives, and feta cheese.

2. In a small bowl, whisk together the olive oil, lemon juice, Dijon mustard, garlic, and dried oregano. Season with salt and pepper to taste.

3. Drizzle the dressing over the salad and toss gently to coat.

4. Serve immediately.

This Greek salad supports the MIND diet for seniors in the following ways:

- Leafy greens like romaine lettuce are a key component of the MIND diet and provide vitamins, minerals, and antioxidants.

- Vegetables like tomatoes, cucumbers, and onions are also emphasized in the MIND diet for their brain-boosting benefits.

- Olives and olive oil are rich in healthy monounsaturated fats, which may help improve cognitive function.

- Feta cheese provides protein and calcium, which are important nutrients for older adults.

- Lemon juice and Dijon mustard in the dressing add a tangy flavor while also providing additional antioxidants.

The MIND diet encourages the consumption of a variety of plant-based foods, and this Greek salad checks all those boxes. It's a refreshing, nutrient-dense meal that can be enjoyed as a main dish or a side salad.

How would you rate this dish?

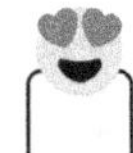 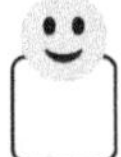  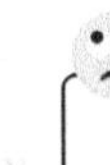 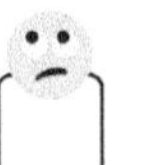 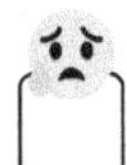

14. Tuna salad with mixed greens and vinaigrette

Let's do that and fill in the time here Prep Time :   Cook Time :   Servings :

Is this dish easy or difficult for you to make?

 ◯   ◯

Write 5 friends with whom you want to share this dish

....

....

....

....

....

INGREDIENTS

Salad:
- 5 cups mixed greens (such as spinach, arugula, and kale)
- 1 (5 oz) can of tuna, drained and flaked
- 1/2 cup cherry tomatoes, halved
- 1/4 cup sliced cucumber
- 2 tablespoons chopped walnuts

Vinaigrette Dressing:
- 2 tablespoons extra-virgin olive oil
- 1 tablespoon balsamic vinegar
- 1 teaspoon Dijon mustard
- 1 teaspoon honey
- 1 garlic clove, minced
- Salt and black pepper to taste

1. In a large salad bowl, combine the mixed greens, tuna, cherry tomatoes, cucumber, and walnuts.

2. In a small bowl, whisk together the olive oil, balsamic vinegar, Dijon mustard, honey, and garlic. Season with salt and pepper to taste.

3. Drizzle the vinaigrette over the salad and toss gently to coat.

4. Serve immediately.

This tuna salad with mixed greens supports the MIND diet for seniors in the following ways:

- Leafy greens like spinach, arugula, and kale are a key component of the MIND diet and provide a variety of vitamins, minerals, and antioxidants.

- Tuna is a good source of lean protein and omega-3 fatty acids, which are important for brain health.

- Walnuts are rich in healthy fats and may help improve cognitive function.

- The vinaigrette dressing is made with olive oil, which is a key component of the MIND diet and provides monounsaturated fats.

- The overall nutrient-dense composition of this salad aligns with the MIND diet's emphasis on whole, plant-based foods.

This tuna salad is a refreshing and satisfying meal that can be enjoyed for lunch or dinner. It's a great option for seniors looking to support their cognitive function and overall health.

How would you rate this dish?

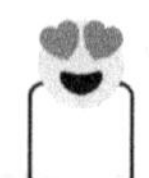 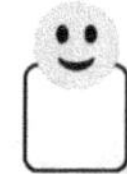  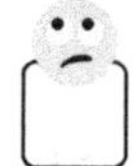 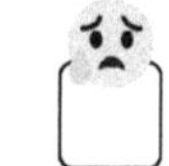

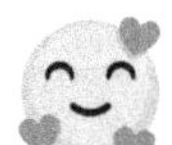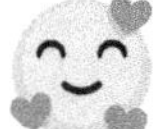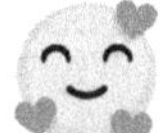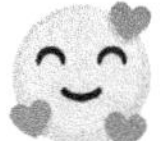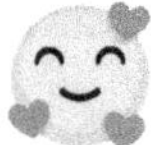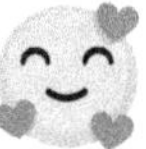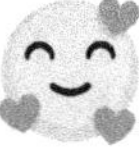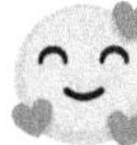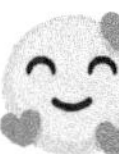

15. Chickpea and spinach curry

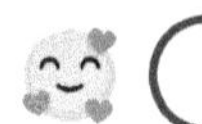 Prep Time :　　　Cook Time :　　　Servings :

Is this dish easy or difficult for you to make?

Write 5 friends with whom you want to share this dish ....

INGREDIENTS

- 1 tablespoon olive oil
- 1 onion, diced
- 3 cloves garlic, minced
- 1 tablespoon grated fresh ginger
- 1 teaspoon ground cumin
- 1 teaspoon ground coriander
- 1/2 teaspoon ground turmeric
- 1/4 teaspoon cayenne pepper (optional)
- 1 (15 oz) can chickpeas, rinsed and drained
- 1 (14 oz) can diced tomatoes
- 1 cup low-sodium vegetable or chicken broth
- 4 cups fresh spinach, chopped
- 1/4 cup chopped fresh cilantro
- Salt and black pepper to taste
- Cooked brown rice, for serving

1. In a large skillet or saucepan, heat the olive oil over medium heat. Add the onion and sauté for 3-4 minutes until translucent.

2. Add the garlic and ginger, and sauté for an additional minute.

3. Stir in the cumin, coriander, turmeric, and cayenne (if using). Cook for 1 minute to toast the spices.

4. Add the chickpeas, diced tomatoes, and broth. Bring the mixture to a simmer and cook for 10-15 minutes, until slightly thickened.

5. Stir in the chopped spinach and cilantro. Cook for 2-3 minutes, until the spinach is wilted.

6. Season the curry with salt and black pepper to taste. Serve the chickpea and spinach curry over cooked brown rice.

This chickpea and spinach curry supports the MIND diet for seniors in the following ways:

- Chickpeas are a legume that provide plant-based protein, fiber, and complex carbs. Spinach is a leafy green vegetable that is rich in vitamins, minerals, and antioxidants.

- Spices like cumin, coriander, and turmeric have anti-inflammatory properties that may benefit brain health. The overall nutrient-dense composition of this curry aligns with the MIND diet's emphasis on whole, plant-based foods.

The combination of protein-rich chickpeas, nutrient-dense spinach, and aromatic spices makes this curry a delicious and nourishing meal for seniors following the MIND diet. Serve it over a bed of whole grain brown rice for added fiber and complex carbs.

How would you rate this dish?

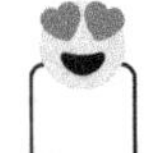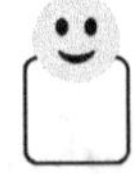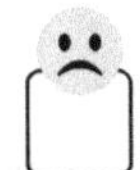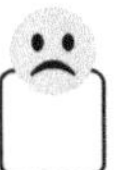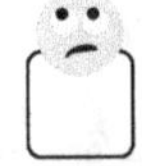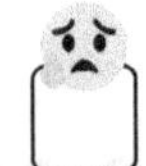

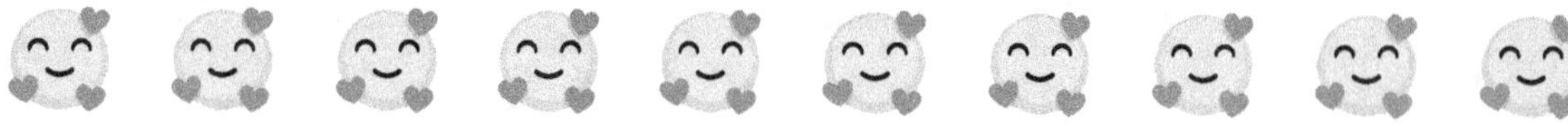

16. Whole-grain wrap with hummus, spinach, and red bell peppers

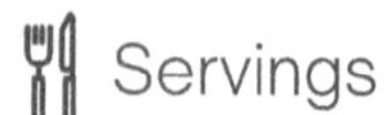 Prep Time :   Cook Time :   Servings :

Is this dish easy or difficult for you to make?

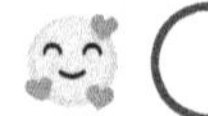 ◯   ◯

Write 5 ....
friends
with   ....
whom
you   ....
want to
share   ....
this
dish   ....

INGREDIENTS

- 1 whole-grain tortilla or wrap
- 2 tablespoons hummus
- 1 cup fresh spinach leaves
- 1/2 red bell pepper, sliced
- 1 tablespoon chopped walnuts (optional)

1. Spread the hummus evenly over the whole-grain tortilla or wrap.

2. Layer the fresh spinach leaves over the hummus.

3. Arrange the sliced red bell pepper on top of the spinach.

4. Sprinkle the chopped walnuts over the vegetables, if using.

5. Carefully roll up the wrap, tucking in the sides as you go. Slice the wrap in half diagonally and serve.

This whole-grain wrap supports the MIND diet for seniors in the following ways:

- Whole-grain tortilla or wrap provides complex carbs, fiber, and B vitamins.
- Hummus is a source of plant-based protein and healthy fats from the tahini and olive oil.
- Spinach is a leafy green vegetable that is rich in vitamins, minerals, and antioxidants.
- Red bell peppers are a colorful vegetable that contains vitamin C and other beneficial plant compounds.
- Walnuts are a good source of omega-3 fatty acids, which are important for brain health.

The MIND diet emphasizes the consumption of whole, plant-based foods, and this wrap checks all those boxes. It's a nutritious and portable option that can be enjoyed for lunch or as a snack.

You can customize the fillings to your liking, such as adding other vegetables or using a different type of nut or seed. The key is to focus on incorporating a variety of nutrient-dense ingredients that support cognitive function and overall health.

How would you rate this dish?

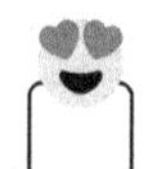 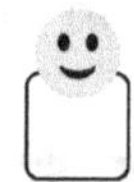 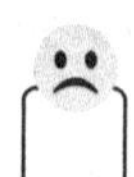 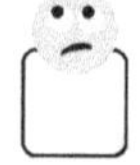 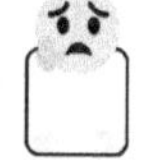

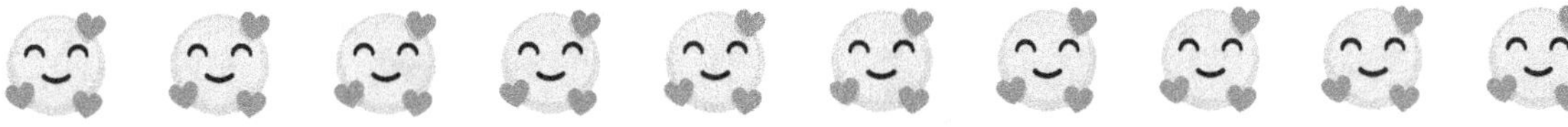

17. Grilled chicken salad with mixed greens and walnuts

Let's do that and fill in the time here  Prep Time :   Cook Time :   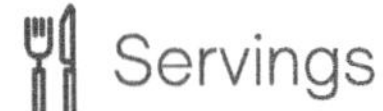 Servings :

Is this dish easy or difficult for you to make?

◯   ◯

Write 5 friends with whom you want to share this dish ....

INGREDIENTS

- 4 oz grilled chicken breast, sliced
- 4 cups mixed greens (such as spinach, arugula, and kale)
- 1/2 cup cherry tomatoes, halved
- 1/4 cup sliced cucumber
- 2 tablespoons chopped walnuts
- 1 tablespoon extra-virgin olive oil
- 1 tablespoon balsamic vinegar
- 1 teaspoon Dijon mustard
- 1 teaspoon honey
- Salt and black pepper to taste

1. In a large salad bowl, combine the grilled chicken, mixed greens, cherry tomatoes, and cucumber.

2. In a small bowl, whisk together the olive oil, balsamic vinegar, Dijon mustard, and honey. Season with salt and pepper to taste.

3. Drizzle the dressing over the salad and toss gently to coat.

4. Sprinkle the chopped walnuts over the top of the salad. Serve immediately.

This grilled chicken salad supports the MIND diet for seniors in the following ways:

- Leafy greens like spinach, arugula, and kale are a key component of the MIND diet and provide a variety of vitamins, minerals, and antioxidants.

- Grilled chicken is a lean protein source that can help maintain muscle mass and strength.

- Walnuts are rich in healthy fats, including omega-3 fatty acids, which are important for brain health.

- The olive oil and balsamic vinegar dressing provides healthy monounsaturated fats and antioxidants.

- The overall nutrient-dense composition of this salad aligns with the MIND diet's emphasis on whole, plant-based foods.

This grilled chicken salad is a refreshing and satisfying meal that can be enjoyed for lunch or dinner. It's a great option for seniors looking to support their cognitive function and overall health while following the MIND diet.

How would you rate this dish?

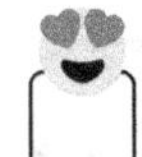 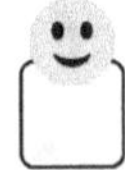  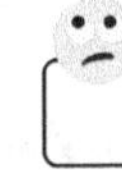 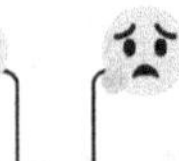

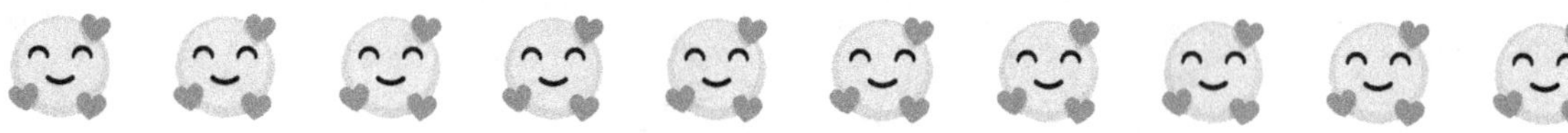

18. Barley and vegetable soup

  Prep Time :   Cook Time :   Servings :

Is this dish easy or difficult for you to make?

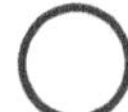 ◯   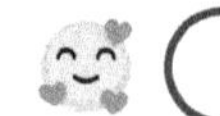 ◯

Write 5 friends with whom you want to share this dish

....

....

....

....

....

INGREDIENTS

- 1 tablespoon olive oil
- 1 onion, diced
- 3 cloves garlic, minced
- 2 carrots, peeled and diced
- 2 celery stalks, diced
- 1 cup pearl barley, rinsed
- 6 cups low-sodium vegetable or chicken broth
- 1 (14.5 oz) can diced tomatoes
- 2 cups chopped kale or spinach
- 1 teaspoon dried thyme
- 1/2 teaspoon dried rosemary
- Salt and black pepper to taste

1. In a large pot or Dutch oven, heat the olive oil over medium heat. Add the onion and sauté for 3-4 minutes until translucent.

2. Add the garlic, carrots, and celery. Sauté for an additional 2-3 minutes.

3. Stir in the pearl barley, broth, diced tomatoes, kale/spinach, thyme, and rosemary. Season with salt and pepper to taste.

4. Bring the soup to a boil, then reduce heat and simmer for 25-30 minutes, or until the barley is tender.

5. Serve hot, garnished with additional chopped kale/spinach if desired.

This barley and vegetable soup supports the MIND diet for seniors in the following ways:

- Barley is a whole grain that provides complex carbs, fiber, and B vitamins.
- Vegetables like carrots, celery, onions, and leafy greens are rich in vitamins, minerals, and antioxidants.
- Herbs like thyme and rosemary have anti-inflammatory properties that may benefit brain health.
- The overall nutrient-dense composition of this soup aligns with the MIND diet's emphasis on whole, plant-based foods.

Barley is a hearty, filling grain that can help seniors feel satisfied and nourished. The combination of vegetables and herbs in this soup provides a variety of beneficial plant compounds to support cognitive function and overall health.

This soup can be enjoyed as a main course or a side dish. It's a comforting and easy-to-prepare meal that can be made in advance and enjoyed throughout the week.

How would you rate this dish?

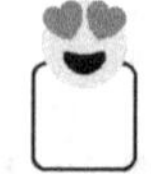 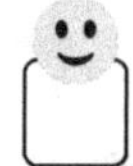 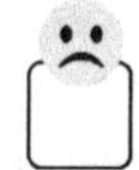 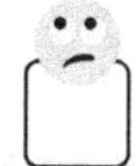 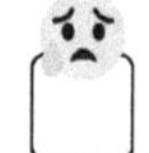

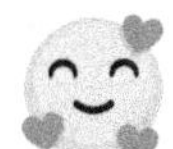 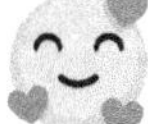 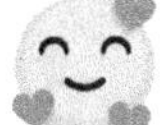 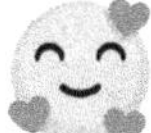 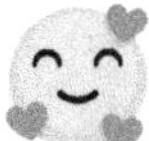 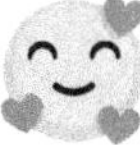 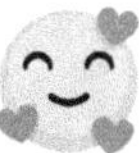 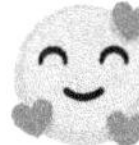 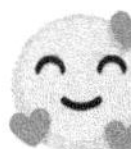 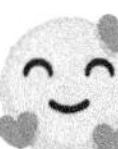

19. Beet and goat cheese salad

Prep Time :   Cook Time :   Servings :

Is this dish easy or difficult for you to make?

Write 5 friends with whom you want to share this dish ....

INGREDIENTS

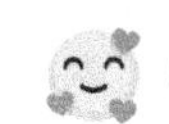

- 3 medium beets, roasted and sliced
- 5 cups mixed greens (such as spinach, arugula, and kale)
- 2 ounces crumbled goat cheese
- 2 tablespoons chopped walnuts
- 2 tablespoons extra-virgin olive oil
- 1 tablespoon balsamic vinegar
- 1 teaspoon Dijon mustard
- 1 teaspoon honey
- Salt and black pepper to taste

1. Preheat your oven to 400°F. Wrap the beets in foil and roast for 45-60 minutes, until tender when pierced with a fork. Allow the beets to cool, then peel and slice them.

2. In a large salad bowl, combine the mixed greens, roasted beet slices, crumbled goat cheese, and chopped walnuts.

3. In a small bowl, whisk together the olive oil, balsamic vinegar, Dijon mustard, and honey. Season with salt and pepper to taste.

4. Drizzle the dressing over the salad and toss gently to coat.

5. Serve the beet and goat cheese salad immediately.

This beet and goat cheese salad supports the MIND diet for seniors in the following ways:

- Leafy greens like spinach, arugula, and kale are a key component of the MIND diet and provide a variety of vitamins, minerals, and antioxidants.
- Beets are a nutrient-dense root vegetable that may help improve cognitive function.
- Goat cheese provides protein and calcium, which are important nutrients for older adults.
- Walnuts are rich in healthy fats, including omega-3 fatty acids, that are beneficial for brain health.
- The olive oil and balsamic vinegar dressing provides healthy monounsaturated fats and antioxidants.

The MIND diet encourages the consumption of a variety of plant-based foods, and this beet and goat cheese salad checks all those boxes. It's a colorful, flavorful, and nutrient-dense meal that can be enjoyed as a main dish or a side salad.

How would you rate this dish?

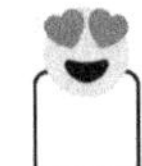 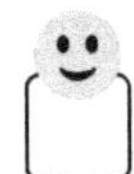 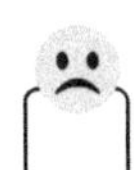 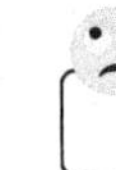 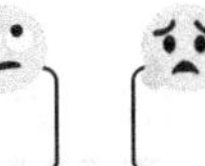 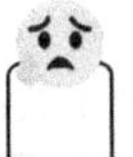

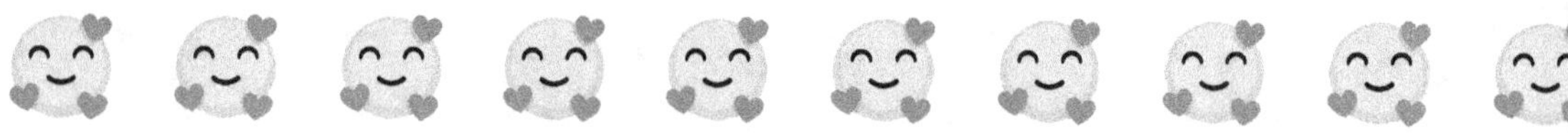

20. Roasted vegetable quinoa bowl

Let's do that and fill in the time here  Prep Time :   Cook Time :   Servings :

Is this dish easy or difficult for you to make?

😭 ◯   🥰 ◯

Write 5 friends with whom you want to share this dish

....

....

....

....

....

INGREDIENTS

- 1 cup uncooked quinoa, rinsed
- 2 cups low-sodium vegetable or chicken broth
- 1 medium sweet potato, peeled and diced
- 1 red bell pepper, diced
- 1 zucchini, diced
- 1 red onion, diced
- 2 tablespoons olive oil
- 1 teaspoon dried thyme
- 1/2 teaspoon dried rosemary
- Salt and black pepper to taste
- 2 cups baby spinach or kale
- 2 tablespoons toasted pumpkin seeds

Dressing:
- 2 tablespoons olive oil
- 1 tablespoon balsamic vinegar
- 1 teaspoon Dijon mustard
- 1 teaspoon honey
- 1 garlic clove, minced
- Salt and black pepper to taste

How would you rate this dish?

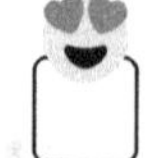 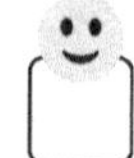 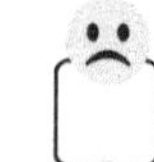 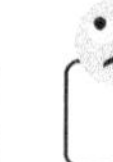 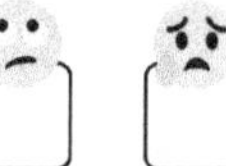

1. Preheat your oven to 400°F. Line a baking sheet with parchment paper.

2. In a large bowl, toss the diced sweet potato, bell pepper, zucchini, and red onion with 2 tablespoons of olive oil, thyme, rosemary, salt, and pepper. Spread the vegetables in a single layer on the prepared baking sheet.

3. Roast the vegetables for 20-25 minutes, stirring halfway, until tender and lightly browned.

4. Meanwhile, in a medium saucepan, combine the quinoa and broth. Bring to a boil, then reduce heat, cover, and simmer for 15-20 minutes, until the quinoa is cooked and the liquid is absorbed.

5. In a small bowl, whisk together the ingredients for the dressing.

6. In a large bowl, combine the cooked quinoa, roasted vegetables, baby spinach/kale, and toasted pumpkin seeds. Drizzle the dressing over the top and toss gently to coat.

7. Serve the roasted vegetable quinoa bowl warm or at room temperature.

This roasted vegetable quinoa bowl supports the MIND diet for seniors in the following ways:

- Quinoa is a whole grain that provides complex carbs, fiber, and protein.
- Roasted vegetables like sweet potato, bell pepper, zucchini, and onion are rich in vitamins, minerals, and antioxidants.
- Leafy greens like spinach and kale are a key component of the MIND diet and provide additional nutrients.
- Pumpkin seeds are a source of healthy fats, including omega-3s, that are important for brain health.

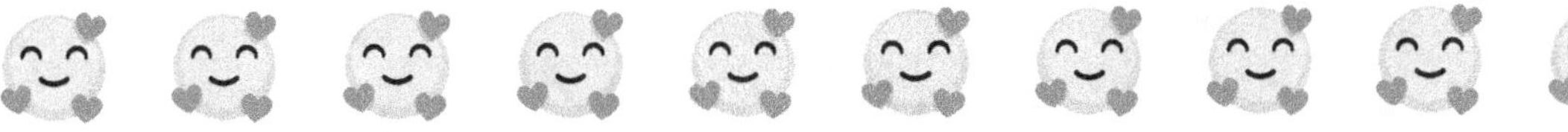

21. Grilled salmon with steamed broccoli

Let's do that and fill in the time here Prep Time :   Cook Time :   Servings :

Is this dish easy or difficult for you to make?

 ◯   ◯

Write 5 friends with whom you want to share this dish ....

INGREDIENTS

- 4 (4 oz) salmon fillets
- 1 tablespoon olive oil
- 1 teaspoon lemon zest
- 1 tablespoon lemon juice
- 1 teaspoon dried dill
- Salt and black pepper to taste
- 4 cups broccoli florets
- 2 tablespoons water

1. Preheat your grill or grill pan to medium-high heat.

2. In a small bowl, mix together the olive oil, lemon zest, lemon juice, and dried dill. Season the salmon fillets with salt and pepper, then brush the top of each fillet with the lemon-dill mixture.

3. Grill the salmon for 4-6 minutes per side, or until it flakes easily with a fork.

4. While the salmon is grilling, place the broccoli florets in a steamer basket and steam for 5-7 minutes, until tender-crisp. Alternatively, you can microwave the broccoli with 2 tablespoons of water for 3-4 minutes. Serve the grilled salmon fillets with the steamed broccoli.

This grilled salmon with steamed broccoli supports the MIND diet for seniors in the following ways:

- Salmon is a fatty fish that is rich in omega-3 fatty acids, which are important for brain health.
- Broccoli is a cruciferous vegetable that is packed with vitamins, minerals, and antioxidants.
- The lemon and dill seasoning provides additional flavor and anti-inflammatory benefits.
- The overall nutrient-dense composition of this meal aligns with the MIND diet's emphasis on whole, plant-based foods and lean protein sources.

Salmon and broccoli are both staples of the MIND diet, as they provide a variety of nutrients that may help protect cognitive function and reduce the risk of age-related cognitive decline.

This grilled salmon and steamed broccoli dish is a simple, yet flavorful and nutritious meal that can be enjoyed by seniors following the MIND diet. It's easy to prepare and can be served with a side of whole grains or a salad for a complete and balanced meal.

How would you rate this dish?

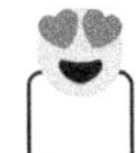 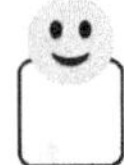 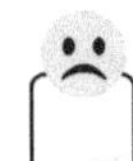 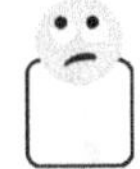 

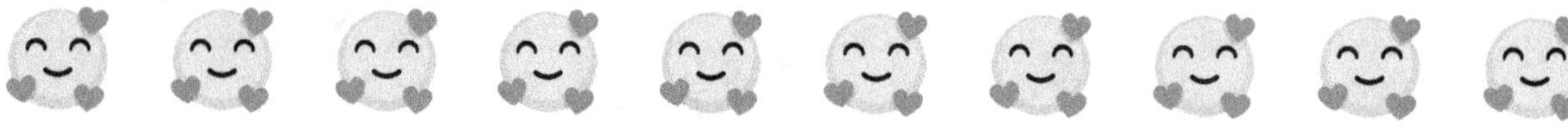

22. Baked chicken breast with sweet potatoes and green beans

 Prep Time :   Cook Time :   Servings :

Is this dish easy or difficult for you to make?

○   ○

Write 5 ....
friends
with ....
whom
you ....
want to
share ....
this
dish ....

INGREDIENTS

- 4 (4 oz) boneless, skinless chicken breasts
- 2 medium sweet potatoes, peeled and diced
- 1 lb green beans, trimmed
- 2 tablespoons olive oil, divided
- 1 teaspoon dried thyme
- 1 teaspoon dried rosemary
- Salt and black pepper to taste

How would you rate this dish?

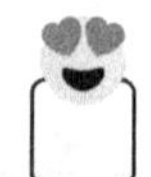 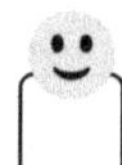 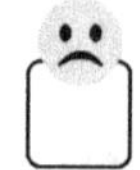 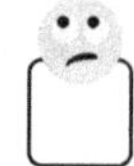 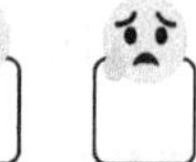 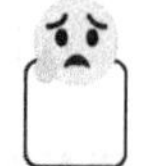

1. Preheat your oven to 400°F. Line a large baking sheet with parchment paper.

2. In a large bowl, toss the diced sweet potatoes with 1 tablespoon of olive oil, thyme, rosemary, salt, and pepper.

3. Spread the seasoned sweet potatoes in a single layer on one side of the prepared baking sheet.

4. In the same bowl, toss the green beans with the remaining 1 tablespoon of olive oil, salt, and pepper.

5. Arrange the green beans in a single layer on the other side of the baking sheet.

6. Place the chicken breasts on the baking sheet, nestled between the sweet potatoes and green beans.

7. Bake for 25-30 minutes, or until the chicken is cooked through (internal temperature reaches 165°F) and the vegetables are tender.

8. Serve the baked chicken breast with the roasted sweet potatoes and green beans.

This baked chicken breast with sweet potatoes and green beans supports the MIND diet for seniors in the following ways:

- Chicken is a lean protein source that can help maintain muscle mass and strength.

- Sweet potatoes are a nutrient-dense root vegetable that are rich in vitamins, minerals, and antioxidants.

- Green beans are a non-starchy vegetable that provides fiber, vitamins, and minerals.

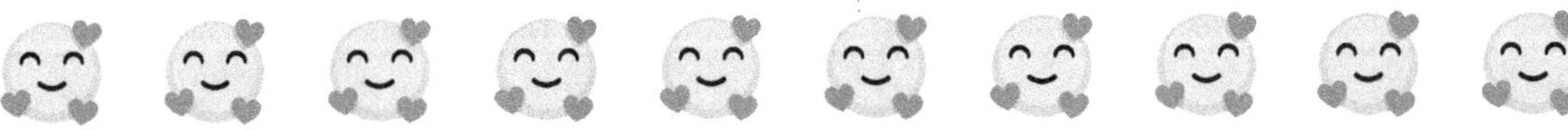

23. Stuffed bell peppers with quinoa and black beans

 Prep Time :   Cook Time :   Servings :

Is this dish easy or difficult for you to make?

Write 5 friends with whom you want to share this dish ....

INGREDIENTS

- 4 bell peppers (any color), halved and seeded
- 1 cup cooked quinoa
- 1 (15 oz) can black beans, rinsed and drained
- 1 cup diced tomatoes
- 1/2 cup crumbled feta cheese
- 2 tablespoons chopped fresh cilantro
- 1 teaspoon ground cumin
- 1/2 teaspoon garlic powder
- Salt and black pepper to taste

How would you rate this dish?

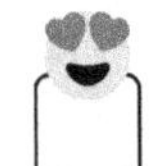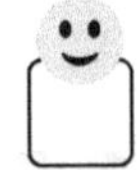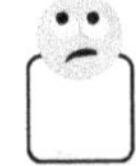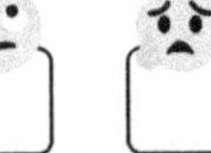

1. Preheat your oven to 375°F. Arrange the bell pepper halves in a baking dish or on a rimmed baking sheet.

2. In a medium bowl, combine the cooked quinoa, black beans, diced tomatoes, feta cheese, cilantro, cumin, and garlic powder. Season with salt and pepper to taste.

3. Spoon the quinoa and black bean mixture evenly into the bell pepper halves.

4. Bake for 25-30 minutes, or until the peppers are tender and the filling is heated through. Serve the stuffed bell peppers warm.

This stuffed bell pepper dish supports the MIND diet for seniors in the following ways:

- Bell peppers are a colorful vegetable that provides vitamins, minerals, and antioxidants. Quinoa is a whole grain that is high in protein, fiber, and complex carbs.

- Black beans are a legume that provide plant-based protein, fiber, and beneficial nutrients.

- Feta cheese is a source of protein and calcium, which are important for older adults. Cilantro and spices like cumin provide anti-inflammatory benefits.

The MIND diet emphasizes the consumption of a variety of plant-based foods, and this stuffed bell pepper recipe checks all those boxes. It's a nutrient-dense and satisfying meal that can be enjoyed as a main dish or a side.

You can customize the filling by using different types of beans, grains, or vegetables to suit your preferences. The key is to focus on incorporating a variety of whole, plant-based ingredients that support cognitive function and overall health.

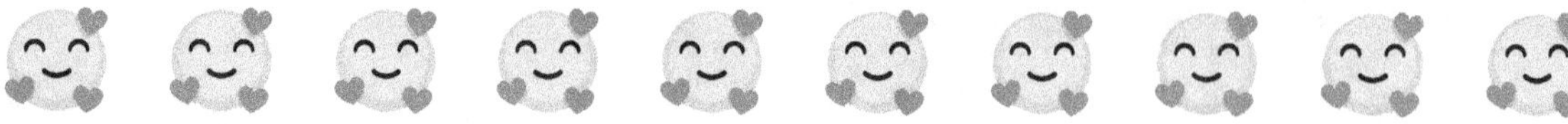

24. Eggplant parmesan with a side of mixed greens

Prep Time :   Cook Time :   Servings :

Is this dish easy or difficult for you to make?

 ○   ○

Write 5 ....
friends
with   ....
whom
you   ....
want to
share ....
this
dish   ....

INGREDIENTS

Eggplant Parmesan:
- 1 medium eggplant, sliced into 1/2-inch rounds
- 1 cup whole-wheat breadcrumbs
- 1/2 cup grated Parmesan cheese
- 2 eggs, beaten
- 1 (24 oz) jar marinara sauce
- 1 cup shredded part-skim mozzarella cheese

Mixed Greens:
- 5 cups mixed greens (such as spinach, arugula, and kale)
- 1 tablespoon extra-virgin olive oil
- 1 tablespoon balsamic vinegar
- Salt and black pepper to taste

Eggplant Parmesan:
1. Preheat your oven to 375°F. Line a baking sheet with parchment paper.
2. In a shallow bowl, combine the breadcrumbs and Parmesan cheese.
3. Dip the eggplant slices in the beaten eggs, then coat them in the breadcrumb mixture.
4. Arrange the breaded eggplant slices in a single layer on the prepared baking sheet.
5. Bake for 20-25 minutes, flipping halfway, until the eggplant is tender and golden brown.
6. Spread a layer of marinara sauce in a baking dish. Arrange the baked eggplant slices on top, then top with the shredded mozzarella cheese.
7. Bake for an additional 15-20 minutes, until the cheese is melted and bubbly.

Mixed Greens:
1. In a large salad bowl, combine the mixed greens.
2. Drizzle the olive oil and balsamic vinegar over the greens, and season with salt and pepper.
3. Toss the salad gently to coat.

Serve the eggplant parmesan warm, with the mixed greens salad on the side.

This eggplant parmesan with mixed greens supports the MIND diet for seniors in the following ways:

- Eggplant is a nutrient-dense vegetable that may have cognitive benefits.
- Whole-wheat breadcrumbs and Parmesan cheese provide a source of protein and complex carbs.
- Leafy greens like spinach, arugula, and kale are a key component of the MIND diet and provide a variety of vitamins, minerals, and antioxidants.
- The olive oil and balsamic vinegar dressing provides healthy monounsaturated fats and antioxidants.

How would you rate this dish?

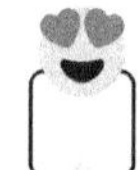 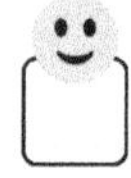 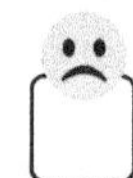 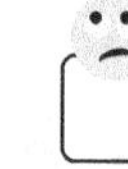 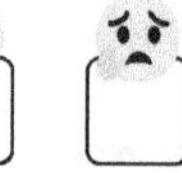

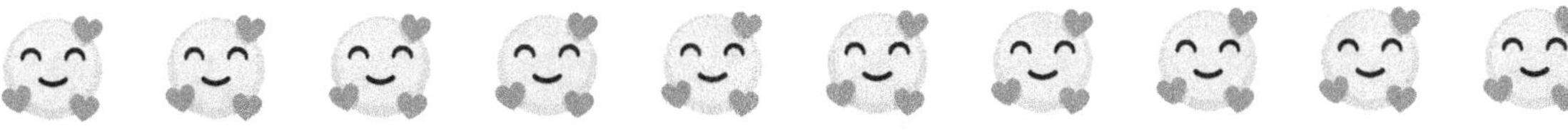

25. Baked cod with a lemon dill sauce and asparagus

Prep Time :   Cook Time :   Servings :

Is this dish easy or difficult for you to make?

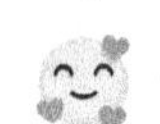 

Write 5 friends with whom you want to share this dish

....

....

....

....

INGREDIENTS

- 4 (4 oz) cod fillets
- 1 lb asparagus, trimmed
- 2 tablespoons olive oil, divided
- Salt and black pepper to taste

Lemon Dill Sauce:
- 1/4 cup plain Greek yogurt
- 2 tablespoons fresh lemon juice
- 1 tablespoon chopped fresh dill
- 1 teaspoon Dijon mustard
- 1 garlic clove, minced
- Salt and black pepper to taste

How would you rate this dish?

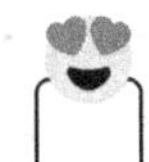 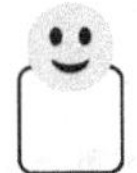 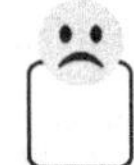 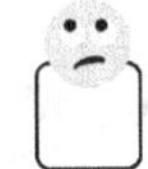 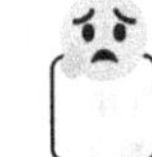

1. Preheat your oven to 400°F. Line a baking sheet with parchment paper.

2. Place the cod fillets and asparagus on the prepared baking sheet. Drizzle 1 tablespoon of olive oil over the cod and asparagus, and season with salt and pepper.

3. Bake for 12-15 minutes, or until the cod is opaque and flakes easily with a fork, and the asparagus is tender-crisp.

Lemon Dill Sauce:
1. In a small bowl, whisk together the Greek yogurt, lemon juice, fresh dill, Dijon mustard, and garlic. Season with salt and pepper to taste.

To Serve: Arrange the baked cod and asparagus on plates. Drizzle the lemon dill sauce over the top of the cod. Serve immediately.

This baked cod with lemon dill sauce and asparagus supports the MIND diet for seniors in the following ways:

- Cod is a lean, flaky fish that is a good source of protein and omega-3 fatty acids, which are important for brain health.
- Asparagus is a nutrient-dense vegetable that provides fiber, vitamins, and antioxidants.
- The lemon dill sauce adds flavor and provides additional antioxidants from the yogurt, lemon, and dill.
- The overall nutrient-dense composition of this dish aligns with the MIND diet's emphasis on whole, plant-based foods and lean protein sources.

This baked cod dish is a simple, yet flavorful and nutritious meal that can be enjoyed by seniors following the MIND diet. The combination of the baked cod, roasted asparagus, and tangy lemon dill sauce creates a well-balanced and satisfying dish.

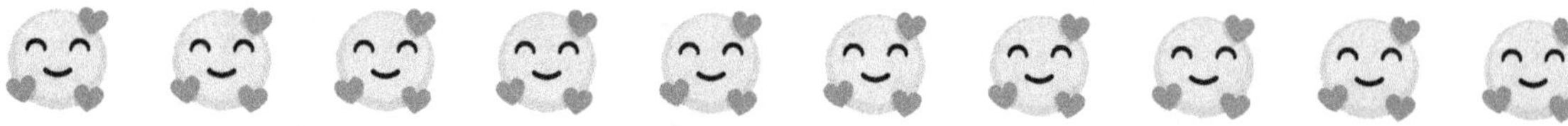

26. Whole-wheat pasta with marinara sauce and sautéed spinach

Prep Time :

Cook Time :

Servings :

Is this dish easy or difficult for you to make?

 ⃝   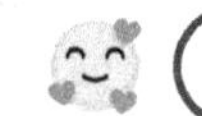 ⃝

Write 5 friends with whom you want to share this dish

....

....

....

....

....

INGREDIENTS

- 8 oz whole-wheat pasta (such as penne or spaghetti)
- 1 tablespoon olive oil
- 3 cloves garlic, minced
- 4 cups fresh spinach, chopped
- 1 (24 oz) jar marinara sauce
- 2 tablespoons grated Parmesan cheese (optional)
- Salt and black pepper to taste

How would you rate this dish?

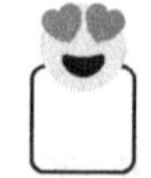 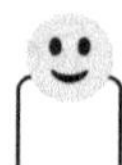 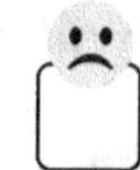 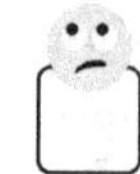 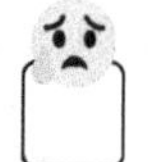

1. Bring a large pot of salted water to a boil. Cook the whole-wheat pasta according to package instructions until al dente. Drain and set aside.

2. In a large skillet, heat the olive oil over medium heat. Add the minced garlic and sauté for 1-2 minutes, until fragrant.

3. Add the chopped spinach to the skillet and sauté for 2-3 minutes, until the spinach is wilted.

4. Pour the marinara sauce into the skillet with the sautéed spinach and garlic. Stir to combine and heat through.

5. Add the cooked whole-wheat pasta to the skillet and toss to coat the pasta evenly with the marinara sauce and spinach.

6. Serve the whole-wheat pasta with marinara and spinach, optionally topped with grated Parmesan cheese.

This whole-wheat pasta dish supports the MIND diet for seniors in the following ways:

- Whole-wheat pasta provides complex carbs, fiber, and B vitamins.
- Spinach is a leafy green vegetable that is rich in vitamins, minerals, and antioxidants.
- Marinara sauce is a plant-based sauce that contains tomatoes, which are a key component of the MIND diet.
- Parmesan cheese provides a source of protein and calcium, which are important nutrients for older adults.

The MIND diet emphasizes the consumption of whole, plant-based foods, and this whole-wheat pasta dish checks all those boxes. It's a comforting and nutritious meal that can be enjoyed by seniors looking to support their cognitive function and overall health

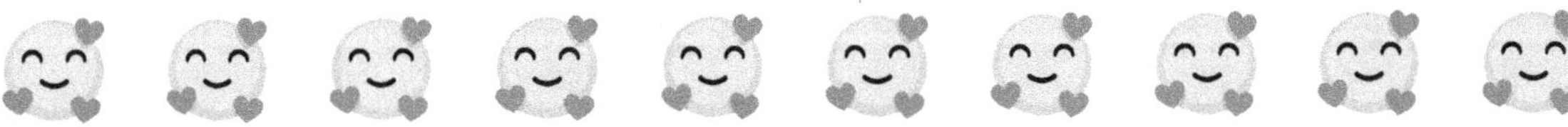

27. Stir-fried tofu with mixed vegetables and brown rice

Is this dish easy or difficult for you to make?

Write 5 friends with whom you want to share this dish ....

INGREDIENTS

- 1 cup uncooked brown rice
- 1 block (14 oz) firm or extra-firm tofu, cubed
- 2 tablespoons low-sodium soy sauce or tamari
- 1 tablespoon sesame oil
- 1 tablespoon rice vinegar
- 1 teaspoon honey
- 2 tablespoons olive oil
- 3 cloves garlic, minced
- 1 inch fresh ginger, peeled and grated
- 2 cups mixed vegetables (such as broccoli, bell peppers, snow peas, and mushrooms), chopped
- 2 tablespoons chopped fresh cilantro (optional)

How would you rate this dish?

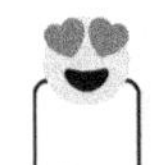 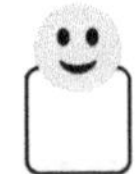 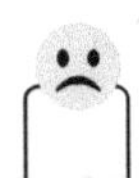 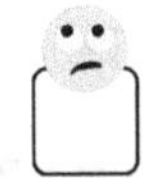 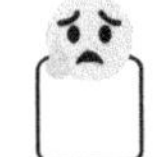

1. Cook the brown rice according to package instructions.

2. In a small bowl, whisk together the soy sauce, sesame oil, rice vinegar, and honey. Set aside.

3. Heat the olive oil in a large skillet or wok over medium-high heat. Add the garlic and ginger and sauté for 1 minute, until fragrant.

4. Add the cubed tofu and stir-fry for 3-4 minutes, until lightly browned on all sides.

5. Add the mixed vegetables to the skillet and continue to stir-fry for 5-7 minutes, until the vegetables are tender-crisp.

6. Pour the soy sauce mixture over the tofu and vegetables and toss to coat everything evenly. Cook for an additional 2-3 minutes, until the sauce has thickened slightly.

7. Serve the stir-fried tofu and vegetables over the cooked brown rice. Garnish with chopped fresh cilantro, if desired.

This stir-fried tofu with mixed vegetables and brown rice supports the MIND diet for seniors in the following ways:

- Tofu is a plant-based protein that provides a lean, cholesterol-free source of protein.
- Brown rice is a whole grain that provides complex carbs, fiber, and B vitamins.
- The mixed vegetables, such as broccoli, bell peppers, and mushrooms, are rich in vitamins, minerals, and antioxidants.
- The soy sauce, sesame oil, and ginger provide additional anti-inflammatory benefits

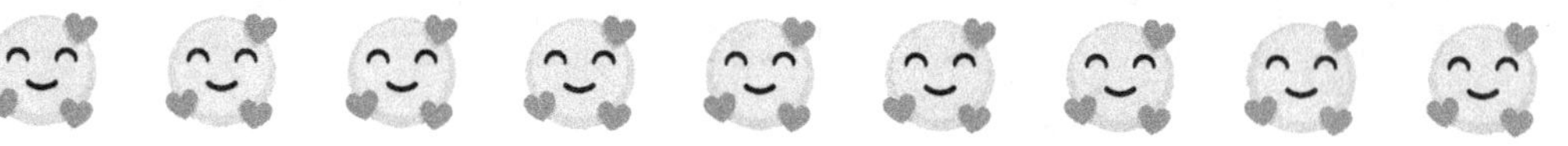

28. Turkey chili with kidney beans

Let's do that and fill in the time here Prep Time :   Cook Time :   Servings :

Is this dish easy or difficult for you to make?

 ◯   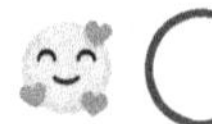 ◯

Write 5 friends with whom you want to share this dish

....

....

....

....

INGREDIENTS

- 1 lb ground turkey
- 1 onion, diced
- 3 cloves garlic, minced
- 2 tablespoons chili powder
- 1 teaspoon ground cumin
- 1 teaspoon dried oregano
- 1/2 teaspoon smoked paprika
- 1/4 teaspoon cayenne pepper (optional)
- 1 (15 oz) can diced tomatoes
- 1 (15 oz) can kidney beans, rinsed and drained
- 1 (15 oz) can black beans, rinsed and drained
- 1 cup low-sodium chicken or vegetable broth
- Salt and black pepper to taste
- Toppings (optional): shredded cheese, diced avocado, chopped cilantro, sour cream

1. In a large pot or Dutch oven, cook the ground turkey over medium-high heat, breaking it up with a wooden spoon, until browned and cooked through, about 5-7 minutes.

2. Add the diced onion and minced garlic to the pot. Sauté for 2-3 minutes, until the onion is translucent.

3. Stir in the chili powder, cumin, oregano, smoked paprika, and cayenne (if using). Cook for 1 minute to toast the spices.

4. Pour in the diced tomatoes, kidney beans, black beans, and chicken/vegetable broth. Stir to combine.

5. Bring the chili to a simmer and let it cook for 20-25 minutes, stirring occasionally, until the flavors have melded and the chili has thickened.

6. Season the chili with salt and black pepper to taste.

7. Serve the turkey chili hot, topped with your desired toppings.

This turkey chili is a hearty, protein-packed meal that can be enjoyed on its own or served with cornbread, tortilla chips, or a side salad. The combination of ground turkey, kidney beans, and spices creates a flavorful and satisfying chili.

Feel free to adjust the spice level by adding more or less cayenne pepper, or swap in different types of beans based on your preferences. This recipe makes a large batch, so you can enjoy leftovers throughout the week.

How would you rate this dish?

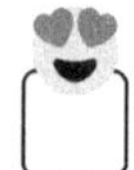 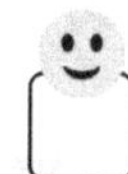 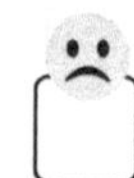 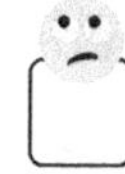 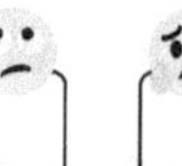 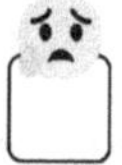

 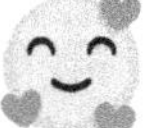  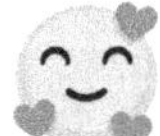 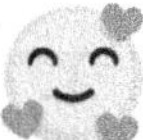 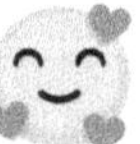 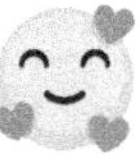   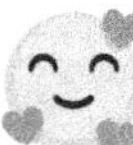

29. Shrimp and vegetable stir-fry

Let's do that and fill in the time here 🕐 Prep Time :   🕐 Cook Time :   🍴 Servings :

Is this dish easy or difficult for you to make?

 ◯    ◯

Write 5 friends with whom you want to share this dish

....
....
....
....
....

INGREDIENTS

- 1 lb shrimp, peeled and deveined
- 2 tablespoons low-sodium soy sauce or tamari
- 1 tablespoon rice vinegar
- 1 teaspoon sesame oil
- 1 tablespoon olive oil
- 3 cloves garlic, minced
- 1 inch fresh ginger, peeled and grated
- 2 cups mixed vegetables (such as broccoli, bell peppers, snow peas, and mushrooms), chopped
- 2 cups cooked brown rice
- 2 tablespoons chopped fresh cilantro (optional)

1. In a small bowl, whisk together the soy sauce, rice vinegar, and sesame oil. Set aside.

2. Heat the olive oil in a large skillet or wok over medium-high heat. Add the minced garlic and grated ginger and sauté for 1 minute, until fragrant.

3. Add the shrimp to the skillet and stir-fry for 2-3 minutes, until the shrimp start to turn pink.

4. Add the mixed vegetables to the skillet and continue to stir-fry for 5-7 minutes, until the vegetables are tender-crisp.

5. Pour the soy sauce mixture over the shrimp and vegetables and toss to coat everything evenly. Cook for an additional 2-3 minutes, until the sauce has thickened slightly.

6. Serve the shrimp and vegetable stir-fry over the cooked brown rice. Garnish with chopped fresh cilantro, if desired.

This shrimp and vegetable stir-fry supports the MIND diet for seniors in the following ways:

- Shrimp is a lean protein source that is rich in omega-3 fatty acids, which are important for brain health.
- The mixed vegetables, such as broccoli, bell peppers, and mushrooms, are rich in vitamins, minerals, and antioxidants.
- Brown rice is a whole grain that provides complex carbs, fiber, and B vitamins.
- The soy sauce, sesame oil, and ginger provide additional anti-inflammatory benefits.
- The overall nutrient-dense composition of this dish aligns with the MIND diet's emphasis on whole, plant-based foods and lean protein sources.

How would you rate this dish?

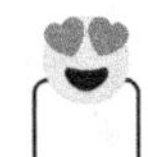 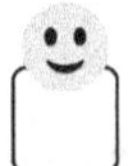 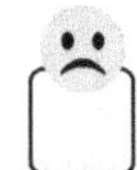 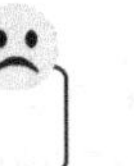 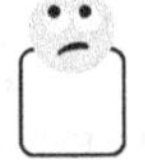 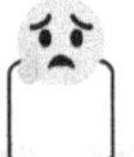

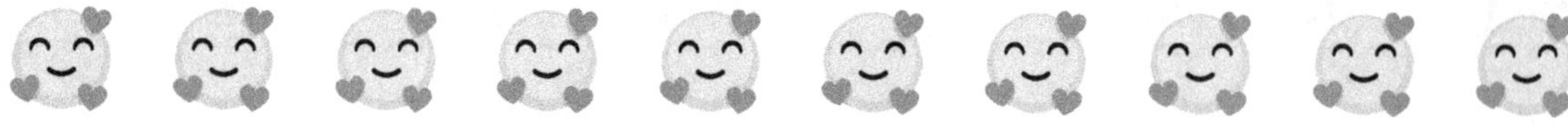

30. Grilled lamb chops with a mint yogurt sauce and roasted vegetables

Prep Time :

Cook Time :

Servings :

Is this dish easy or difficult for you to make?

 ○   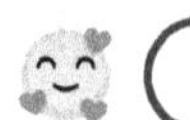 ○

Write 5 friends with whom you want to share this dish

....

....

....

....

....

INGREDIENTS

- 8 lamb chops, about 1-inch thick
- 2 tbsp olive oil
- Salt and pepper to taste
- 1 cup plain Greek yogurt
- 1/4 cup chopped fresh mint
- 1 tbsp lemon juice
- 1 tsp honey
- 3 cups mixed vegetables (such as carrots, zucchini, bell peppers), cut into 1-inch pieces
- 2 tbsp olive oil
- Salt and pepper to taste

1. Preheat grill or grill pan to medium-high heat.

2. Season the lamb chops with salt and pepper on both sides. Drizzle with 2 tbsp olive oil.

3. Grill the lamb chops for 3-4 minutes per side, or until they reach your desired doneness. Transfer to a plate and let rest for 5 minutes.

4. In a small bowl, mix together the yogurt, mint, lemon juice, and honey. Season with salt and pepper to taste.

5. Toss the mixed vegetables with 2 tbsp olive oil and season with salt and pepper.

6. Spread the vegetables out on a baking sheet and roast at 400°F for 20-25 minutes, stirring halfway, until tender and lightly browned.

7. Serve the grilled lamb chops with the mint yogurt sauce and the roasted vegetables on the side.

Enjoy your delicious and healthy grilled lamb chops meal!

How would you rate this dish?

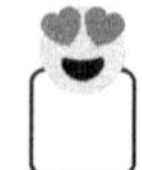 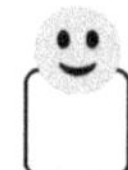 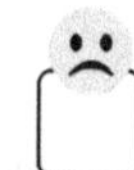 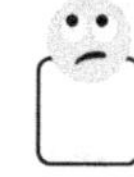 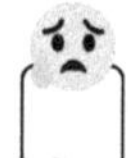

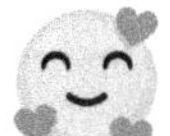 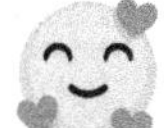 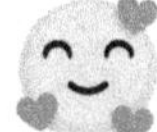 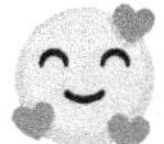  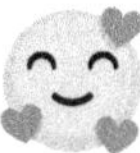 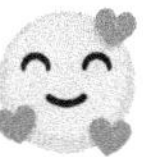 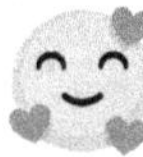 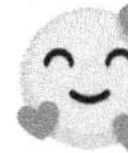 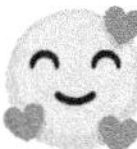

31. Mixed nuts (walnuts, almonds, pecans)

Let's do that and fill in the time here   Prep Time :   Cook Time :   Servings :

Is this dish easy or difficult for you to make?

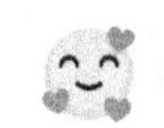

Write 5 friends with whom you want to share this dish

....

....

....

....

....

INGREDIENTS

- 1 cup raw walnuts
- 1 cup raw almonds
- 1 cup raw pecans
- 1 tsp ground cinnamon
- 1/2 tsp ground ginger
- 1/4 tsp sea salt

1. Preheat the oven to 325°F.

2. In a large bowl, combine the walnuts, almonds, and pecans.

3. Sprinkle the cinnamon, ginger, and salt over the nuts and toss to coat evenly.

4. Spread the seasoned nuts out in a single layer on a baking sheet.

5. Roast for 10-12 minutes, stirring halfway, until the nuts are lightly toasted and fragrant.

6. Allow the nuts to cool completely before serving.

7. Store the mixed nuts in an airtight container at room temperature for up to 2 weeks.

This mix of walnuts, almonds, and pecans provides a variety of healthy fats, protein, fiber, and antioxidants that are beneficial for brain health, especially for seniors following the MIND diet. The cinnamon and ginger add extra flavor and anti-inflammatory properties.

Enjoy this nutritious and delicious mixed nuts snack as part of a balanced MIND diet meal plan.

How would you rate this dish?

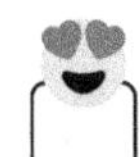 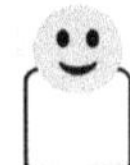 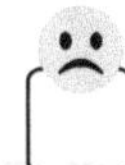 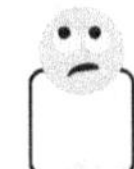 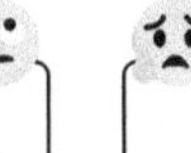

32. Apple slices with almond butter

 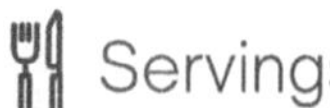

Prep Time :   Cook Time :   Servings :

Is this dish easy or difficult for you to make?

Write 5 friends with whom you want to share this dish ....

INGREDIENTS

- 2 medium apples, cored and sliced
- 1/4 cup all-natural almond butter
- 1 tbsp honey (optional)
- 1/4 tsp ground cinnamon

1. Wash and slice the apples into thin wedges or slices.

2. In a small bowl, stir together the almond butter and honey (if using) until well combined.

3. Arrange the apple slices on a plate or platter.

4. Drizzle or spoon the almond butter mixture over the apple slices, making sure to coat them evenly.

5. Sprinkle the ground cinnamon over the top.

That's it! This simple snack is a great way to incorporate the MIND diet principles:

- Apples are a good source of fiber, antioxidants, and flavonoids that support brain health.

- Almond butter provides healthy fats, protein, and vitamin E, which are important for cognitive function.

- Cinnamon is an anti-inflammatory spice that may help improve memory and cognitive abilities.

This snack is easy to prepare, portable, and satisfying. It makes a great mid-afternoon pick-me-up or a healthy dessert option for seniors following the MIND diet.

Enjoy this delicious and nutritious apple and almond butter treat!

How would you rate this dish?

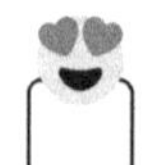 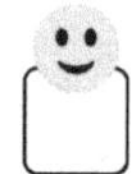 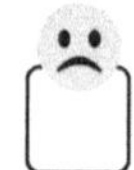 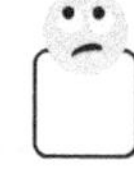 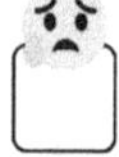

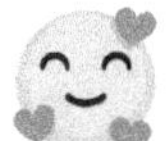 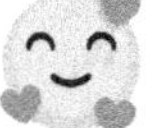 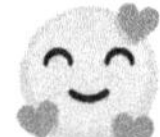 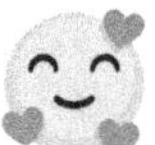 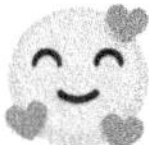 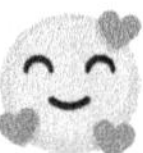 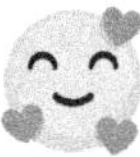 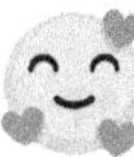  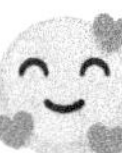

33. Carrot sticks with hummus

Let's do that and fill in the time here 🕐 Prep Time :   🕐 Cook Time :   🍴 Servings :

Is this dish easy or difficult for you to make?

😱 ◯   😊 ◯

Write 5 friends with whom you want to share this dish
....
....
....
....
....

INGREDIENTS

- 4-5 medium carrots, peeled and cut into sticks
- 1 cup homemade or store-bought hummus

1. Wash and peel the carrots. Cut them into long, thin sticks, about 4-5 inches long.

2. Place the carrot sticks in a serving bowl or plate.

3. Scoop the hummus into a small bowl or ramekin and place it next to the carrot sticks.

That's it! This simple snack is a great way to incorporate the MIND diet principles:

- Carrots are a rich source of beta-carotene, fiber, and antioxidants, which are beneficial for brain health.

- Hummus is made from chickpeas, which are a good source of protein, fiber, and complex carbohydrates. The tahini (sesame seed paste) in hummus also provides healthy fats.

This snack is easy to prepare, portable, and satisfying. It makes a great mid-afternoon pick-me-up or a healthy snack option for seniors following the MIND diet.

The combination of the crunchy, nutrient-dense carrots and the creamy, protein-rich hummus provides a balanced and delicious way to support cognitive function and overall brain health.

Enjoy this simple yet nourishing carrot and hummus snack!

How would you rate this dish?

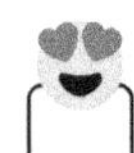 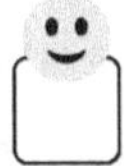 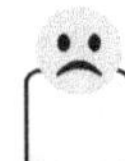 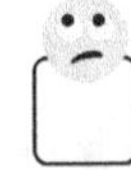 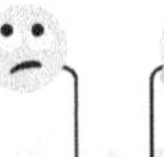

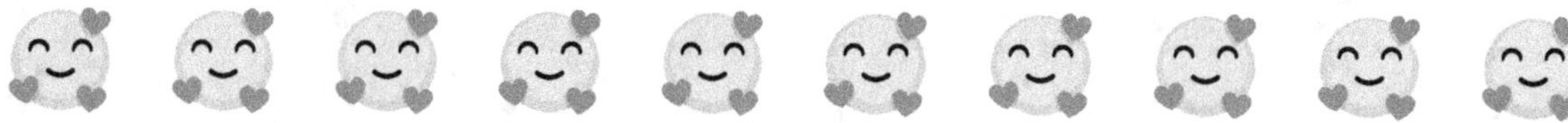

34. Fresh berries with a handful of sunflower seeds

 Prep Time :   Cook Time :   Servings :

Is this dish easy or difficult for you to make?

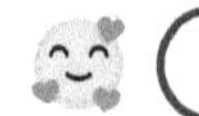 ⭕   ⭕

Write 5 ....
friends
with ....
whom
you ....
want to
share ....
this
dish ....

INGREDIENTS

- 1 cup mixed fresh berries (such as blueberries, raspberries, blackberries)
- 2 tablespoons raw, unsalted sunflower seeds

1. Rinse the fresh berries and gently pat them dry with a paper towel.

2. Place the berries in a small bowl or plate.

3. Sprinkle the raw sunflower seeds over the top of the berries.

That's it! This simple snack is a great way to incorporate the MIND diet principles:

- Berries are rich in antioxidants, flavonoids, and other nutrients that are beneficial for brain health. They have been shown to improve cognitive function and memory.
- Sunflower seeds are a good source of healthy fats, protein, fiber, and vitamins like vitamin E, which is important for brain health.

This snack is easy to prepare, portable, and satisfying. It makes a great mid-afternoon pick-me-up or a healthy dessert option for seniors following the MIND diet.

The combination of the sweet, juicy berries and the crunchy, nutrient-dense sunflower seeds provides a balanced and delicious way to support cognitive function and overall brain health.

Enjoy this simple yet nourishing berry and sunflower seed snack!

How would you rate this dish?

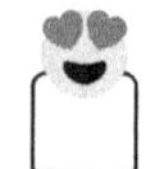 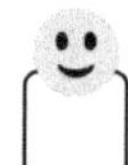  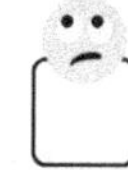 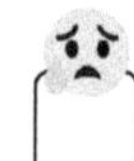 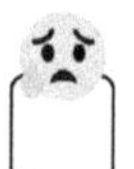

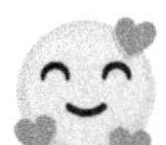 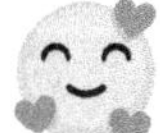 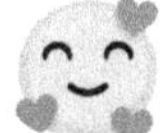 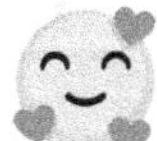 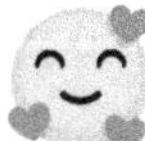 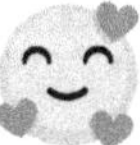 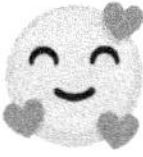   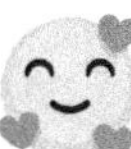

35. Air-popped popcorn with olive oil

Is this dish easy or difficult for you to make?

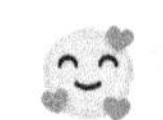

Write 5 friends with whom you want to share this dish ....

INGREDIENTS

- 1/2 cup unpopped popcorn kernels
- 1 tablespoon extra-virgin olive oil
- 1/4 teaspoon sea salt (optional)

1. In an air popper, pop the popcorn kernels according to the manufacturer's instructions.

2. Once the popping is complete, transfer the air-popped popcorn to a large bowl.

3. Drizzle the olive oil over the popcorn and gently toss to coat evenly.

4. If desired, sprinkle the sea salt over the popcorn and toss again to distribute.

That's it! This simple snack is a great way to incorporate the MIND diet principles:

- Air-popped popcorn is a whole grain that provides fiber, which is important for brain health.

- Olive oil is a healthy monounsaturated fat that has been shown to have anti-inflammatory properties and may help improve cognitive function.

- The sea salt (if used) provides a small amount of sodium, which is necessary for proper brain function.

This snack is easy to prepare, low in calories, and satisfying. It makes a great mid-afternoon pick-me-up or a healthy snack option for seniors following the MIND diet.

The combination of the crunchy, whole-grain popcorn and the heart-healthy olive oil provides a balanced and delicious way to support cognitive function and overall brain health.

Enjoy this simple yet nourishing air-popped popcorn with olive oil!

How would you rate this dish?

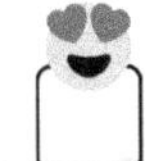 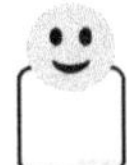 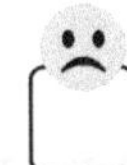 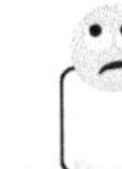 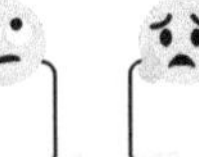

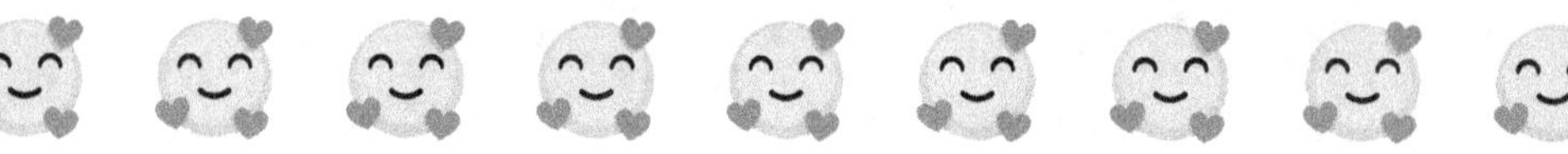

36. Whole-grain crackers with guacamole

 Prep Time :   Cook Time :   Servings :

Is this dish easy or difficult for you to make?

 ◯   ◯

Write 5 friends with whom you want to share this dish

....

....

....

....

....

INGREDIENTS

- 1 ripe avocado
- 1 tablespoon fresh lime juice
- 2 tablespoons diced red onion
- 1 tablespoon chopped cilantro (optional)
- 1/4 teaspoon sea salt
- 1/8 teaspoon ground cumin
- 12-15 whole-grain crackers

1. In a medium bowl, mash the avocado with a fork until it reaches your desired consistency.

2. Add the lime juice, red onion, cilantro (if using), sea salt, and cumin. Stir to combine.

3. Taste the guacamole and adjust seasoning as needed.

4. Serve the guacamole with the whole-grain crackers.

This snack is a great way to incorporate the MIND diet principles:

- Whole-grain crackers provide complex carbohydrates, fiber, and other nutrients that are important for brain health.

- Avocado is a rich source of healthy monounsaturated fats, which have been shown to improve cognitive function and reduce the risk of Alzheimer's disease.

- The lime juice, onion, and cilantro add antioxidants and anti-inflammatory compounds to the guacamole.

This snack is easy to prepare, portable, and satisfying. It makes a great mid-afternoon pick-me-up or a healthy snack option for seniors following the MIND diet.

The combination of the crunchy, whole-grain crackers and the creamy, nutrient-dense guacamole provides a balanced and delicious way to support cognitive function and overall brain health.

Enjoy this simple yet nourishing whole-grain crackers with guacamole snack!

How would you rate this dish?

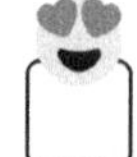 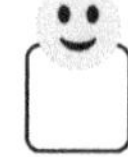 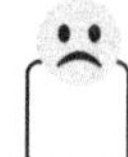  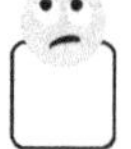 

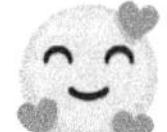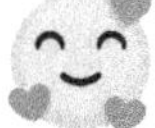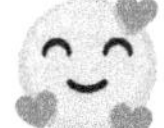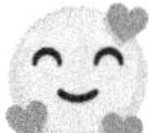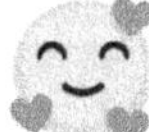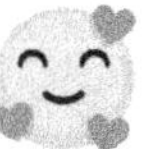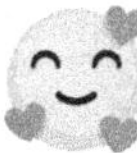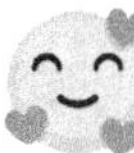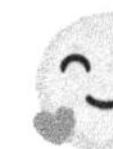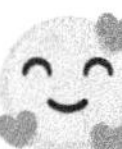

37. Edamame with sea salt

Let's do that and fill in the time here 🕐 Prep Time :   🕐 Cook Time :   🍴 Servings :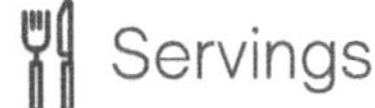

Is this dish easy or difficult for you to make?

○   ○

Write 5 friends with whom you want to share this dish

....

....

....

....

....

INGREDIENTS

- 1 pound frozen edamame in the pod
- 1 teaspoon sea salt

1. Bring a large pot of water to a boil.

2. Add the frozen edamame pods to the boiling water and cook for 5-7 minutes, or until the pods are tender.

3. Drain the edamame and transfer them to a serving bowl.

4. Sprinkle the sea salt over the hot edamame and toss to coat evenly.

5. Serve the edamame warm, with the pods still intact.

This simple snack is a great way to incorporate the MIND diet principles:

- Edamame is a soy-based food that is rich in protein, fiber, and antioxidants, all of which are important for brain health.
- Sea salt provides a small amount of sodium, which is necessary for proper brain function.

This snack is easy to prepare, portable, and satisfying. It makes a great mid-afternoon pick-me-up or a healthy snack option for seniors following the MIND diet.

The combination of the protein-rich edamame and the simple seasoning of sea salt provides a balanced and delicious way to support cognitive function and overall brain health.

Edamame is also a good source of folate, which is a nutrient that has been linked to a reduced risk of Alzheimer's disease and other forms of dementia.

Enjoy this simple yet nourishing edamame with sea salt snack!

How would you rate this dish?

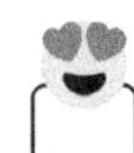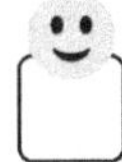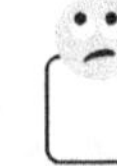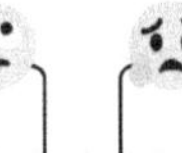

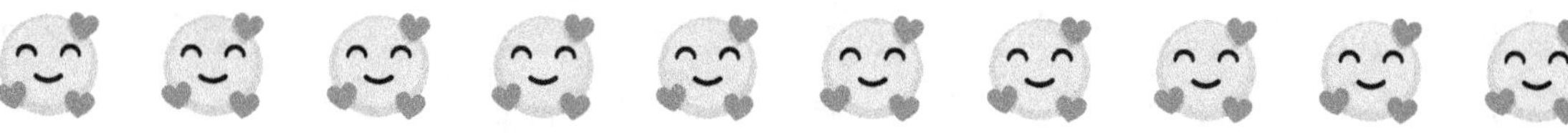

38. Greek yogurt with a drizzle of honey

Prep Time :   Cook Time :   Servings :

Is this dish easy or difficult for you to make?

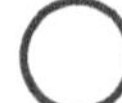 ○    ○

Write 5 ....
friends
with ....
whom
you ....
want to
share ....
this
dish ....

INGREDIENTS

- 1 cup plain Greek yogurt
- 1-2 tablespoons raw, unprocessed honey

1. Scoop the Greek yogurt into a serving bowl or cup.

2. Drizzle the honey over the top of the yogurt.

That's it! This simple snack is a great way to incorporate the MIND diet principles:

- Greek yogurt is a rich source of protein, which is important for brain health and cognitive function.
- Honey is a natural sweetener that contains antioxidants and anti-inflammatory compounds, which may help protect the brain.

This snack is easy to prepare, portable, and satisfying. It makes a great mid-afternoon pick-me-up or a healthy dessert option for seniors following the MIND diet.

The combination of the creamy, protein-rich Greek yogurt and the sweet, nutrient-dense honey provides a balanced and delicious way to support cognitive function and overall brain health.

You can also try adding a sprinkle of cinnamon or a handful of fresh berries to this snack for an extra boost of brain-healthy nutrients.

Enjoy this simple yet nourishing Greek yogurt with honey!

How would you rate this dish?

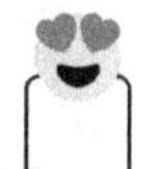 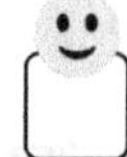  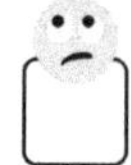 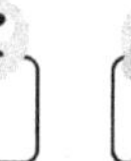 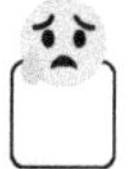

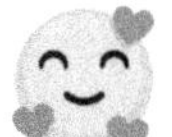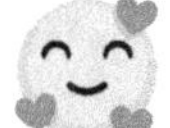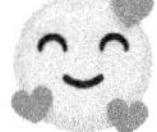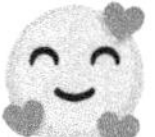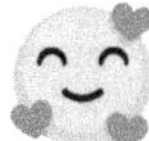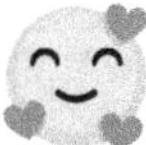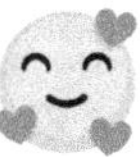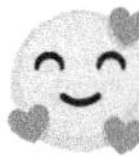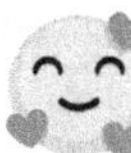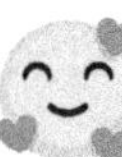

39. Cottage cheese with pineapple chunks

Let's do that and fill in the time here 🕐 Prep Time :   🕐 Cook Time :   🍴 Servings :

Is this dish easy or difficult for you to make?

Write 5 friends with whom you want to share this dish

....
....
....
....
....

INGREDIENTS

- 1 cup low-fat or non-fat cottage cheese
- 1/2 cup fresh pineapple chunks
- 1 teaspoon honey (optional)

1. Scoop the cottage cheese into a serving bowl or cup.

2. Top the cottage cheese with the fresh pineapple chunks.

3. If desired, drizzle the honey over the top of the pineapple and cottage cheese.

This simple snack is a great way to incorporate the MIND diet principles:

- Cottage cheese is a good source of protein, which is important for brain health and cognitive function.

- Pineapple is rich in vitamin C, manganese, and bromelain, which are all beneficial for brain function and reducing inflammation.

- The optional honey provides a natural sweetener with antioxidant properties.

This snack is easy to prepare, portable, and satisfying. It makes a great mid-afternoon pick-me-up or a healthy snack option for seniors following the MIND diet.

The combination of the creamy, protein-rich cottage cheese and the sweet, juicy pineapple chunks provides a balanced and delicious way to support cognitive function and overall brain health.

You can also try adding a sprinkle of cinnamon or a handful of chopped nuts for an extra boost of brain-healthy nutrients.

Enjoy this simple yet nourishing cottage cheese with pineapple snack!

How would you rate this dish?

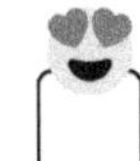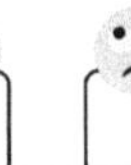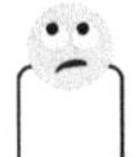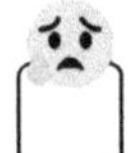

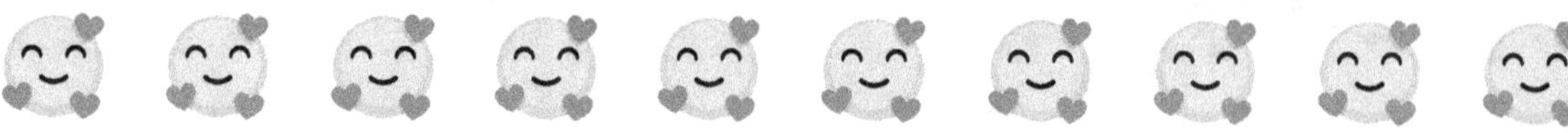

40. Dark chocolate squares

Let's do that and fill in the time here   Prep Time :   Cook Time :   Servings :

Is this dish easy or difficult for you to make?

 ◯   ◯

Write 5 friends with whom you want to share this dish

....

....

....

....

....

INGREDIENTS

- 1 ounce (1-2 squares) of high-quality dark chocolate (70% cacao or higher)

1. Break off 1-2 squares of the dark chocolate.

2. Savor the dark chocolate slowly, allowing it to melt in your mouth.

This simple snack is a great way to incorporate the MIND diet principles:

- Dark chocolate is rich in flavonoids, which are antioxidants that have been shown to improve cognitive function and reduce the risk of Alzheimer's disease.

- The high cacao content in dark chocolate (70% or higher) provides a concentrated source of these beneficial flavonoids.

This snack is easy to prepare, portable, and satisfying. It makes a great mid-afternoon pick-me-up or a healthy dessert option for seniors following the MIND diet.

The rich, intense flavor of the dark chocolate can help satisfy sweet cravings while providing a boost of brain-healthy nutrients.

It's important to keep the portion size small, as dark chocolate is still high in calories and fat. Stick to 1-2 squares per serving to reap the benefits without overindulging.

Enjoy this simple yet indulgent dark chocolate square snack as part of a balanced MIND diet meal plan.

How would you rate this dish?

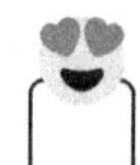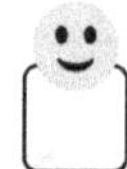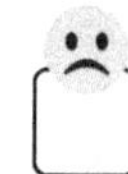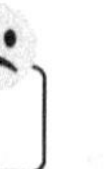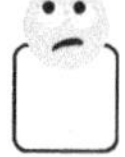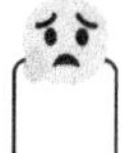

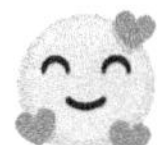 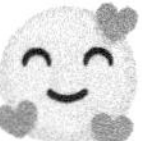 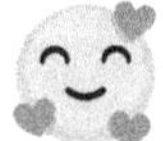 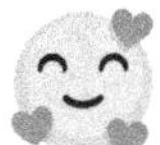 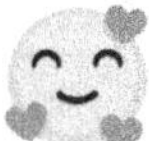 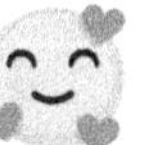 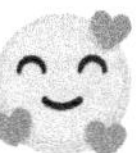 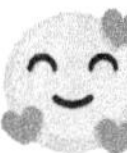  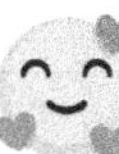

41. Tomato basil soup

Prep Time :   Cook Time :   Servings :

Is this dish easy or difficult for you to make?

 ◯   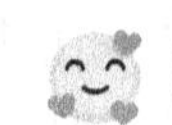 ◯

Write 5 friends with whom you want to share this dish

....

....

....

....

....

INGREDIENTS

- 2 tablespoons olive oil
- 1 onion, diced
- 3 cloves garlic, minced
- 2 (28-ounce) cans diced tomatoes
- 2 cups low-sodium vegetable or chicken broth
- 1/4 cup fresh basil leaves, chopped
- 1 teaspoon dried oregano
- 1/4 teaspoon red pepper flakes (optional)
- Salt and black pepper to taste
- 2 tablespoons grated Parmesan cheese (optional)

1. In a large pot or Dutch oven, heat the olive oil over medium heat. Add the diced onion and sauté for 5-7 minutes, until translucent.

2. Add the minced garlic and sauté for an additional 1-2 minutes, until fragrant.

3. Pour in the canned diced tomatoes and the broth. Bring the mixture to a simmer.

4. Stir in the chopped fresh basil, dried oregano, and red pepper flakes (if using). Season with salt and black pepper to taste.

5. Reduce the heat to low and let the soup simmer for 15-20 minutes, allowing the flavors to meld.

6. Serve the tomato basil soup hot, garnished with a sprinkle of grated Parmesan cheese (if desired).

This soup is a great way to incorporate the MIND diet principles:

- Tomatoes are a rich source of lycopene, an antioxidant that has been linked to improved cognitive function.

- Basil is an anti-inflammatory herb that may help protect the brain.

- Olive oil provides healthy monounsaturated fats that are beneficial for brain health.

This soup is easy to prepare, comforting, and satisfying. It makes a great lunch or dinner option for seniors following the MIND diet.

Enjoy this delicious and nutritious tomato basil soup!

How would you rate this dish?

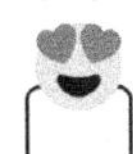 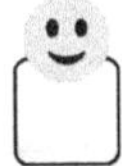 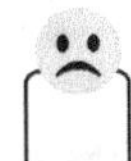 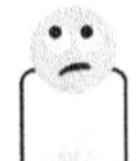 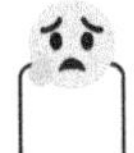

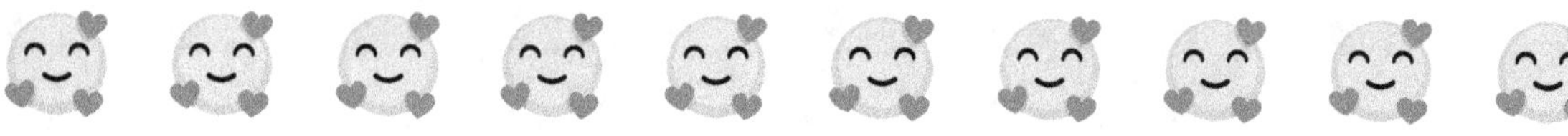

42. Minestrone soup with whole-grain pasta

Let's do that and fill in the time here ✓ Prep Time :   ⏱ Cook Time :   🍴 Servings :

Is this dish easy or difficult for you to make?

 ◯   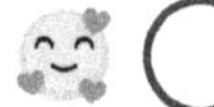 ◯

Write 5 friends with whom you want to share this dish

....
....
....
....
....

INGREDIENTS

- 2 tablespoons olive oil
- 1 onion, diced
- 3 carrots, peeled and diced
- 2 celery stalks, diced
- 3 cloves garlic, minced
- 1 (15-ounce) can diced tomatoes
- 4 cups low-sodium vegetable or chicken broth
- 1 (15-ounce) can kidney beans, rinsed and drained
- 1 cup chopped kale or spinach
- 1/2 cup whole-grain elbow macaroni or small pasta shapes
- 2 tablespoons chopped fresh basil
- Salt and black pepper to taste
- Grated Parmesan cheese (optional)

1. In a large pot or Dutch oven, heat the olive oil over medium heat. Add the diced onion, carrots, and celery. Sauté for 5-7 minutes, until the vegetables are softened.

2. Add the minced garlic and sauté for an additional 1-2 minutes, until fragrant.

3. Pour in the canned diced tomatoes and the broth. Bring the mixture to a simmer.

4. Stir in the rinsed and drained kidney beans, chopped kale or spinach, and the whole-grain pasta.

5. Reduce the heat to low and let the soup simmer for 15-20 minutes, or until the pasta is tender.

6. Remove from heat and stir in the chopped fresh basil. Season with salt and black pepper to taste.

7. Serve the minestrone soup hot, garnished with grated Parmesan cheese (if desired).

This soup is a great way to incorporate the MIND diet principles:

- Whole-grain pasta provides complex carbohydrates, fiber, and other nutrients that are important for brain health.

- Vegetables like carrots, celery, and kale/spinach are rich in antioxidants and other brain-boosting compounds.

- Kidney beans are a good source of protein, fiber, and folate, which are all beneficial for cognitive function.

This soup is easy to prepare, comforting, and satisfying. It makes a great lunch or dinner option for seniors following the MIND diet.

How would you rate this dish?

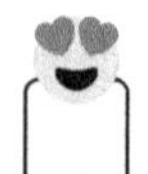 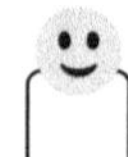 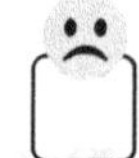 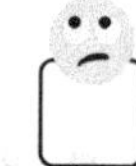 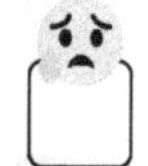

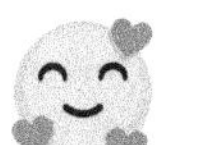 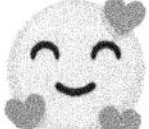 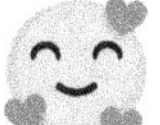 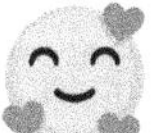 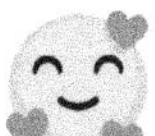 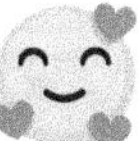 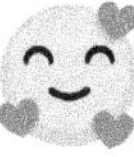 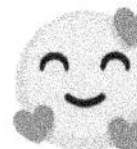 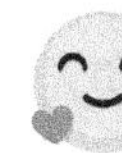 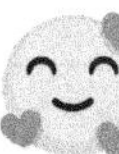

43. Butternut squash soup

  Prep Time :   Cook Time :   Servings :

Is this dish easy or difficult for you to make?

 ◯   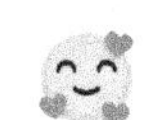 ◯

Write 5 friends with whom you want to share this dish

....

....

....

....

....

INGREDIENTS

- 1 medium butternut squash, peeled, seeded, and cubed (about 4 cups)
- 1 onion, diced
- 2 cloves garlic, minced
- 2 cups low-sodium vegetable or chicken broth
- 1 cup unsweetened almond milk (or regular milk)
- 1 teaspoon ground cinnamon
- 1/4 teaspoon ground nutmeg
- Salt and black pepper to taste
- Chopped fresh parsley or thyme for garnish (optional)

1. In a large pot or Dutch oven, sauté the diced onion in a small amount of olive oil over medium heat for 5-7 minutes, until translucent.

2. Add the minced garlic and sauté for an additional 1-2 minutes, until fragrant.

3. Add the cubed butternut squash, broth, and almond milk (or regular milk) to the pot. Bring the mixture to a simmer.

4. Reduce the heat to low, cover the pot, and let the soup simmer for 20-25 minutes, or until the squash is very soft.

5. Using an immersion blender or a regular blender, puree the soup until smooth and creamy.

6. Stir in the ground cinnamon and nutmeg. Season with salt and black pepper to taste.

7. Serve the butternut squash soup hot, garnished with chopped fresh parsley or thyme (if desired).

This soup is a great way to incorporate the MIND diet principles:

- Butternut squash is a rich source of beta-carotene, an antioxidant that has been linked to improved cognitive function.

- Cinnamon and nutmeg are spices that have anti-inflammatory properties and may help protect the brain.

- The almond milk (or regular milk) provides a creamy texture and a boost of protein.

This soup is easy to prepare, comforting, and satisfying. It makes a great lunch or dinner option for seniors following the MIND diet

How would you rate this dish?

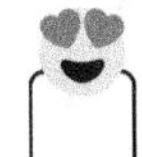 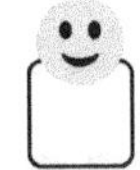 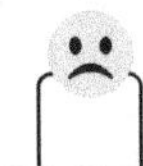 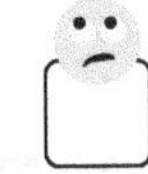 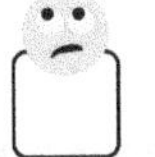 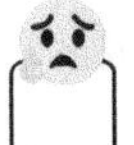

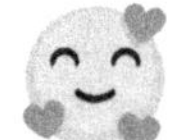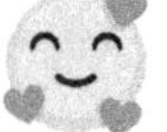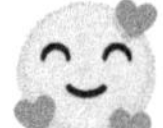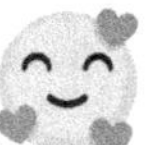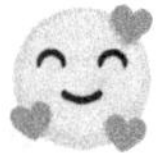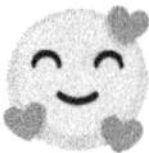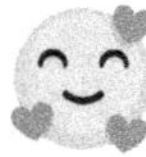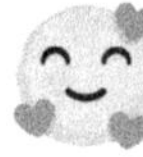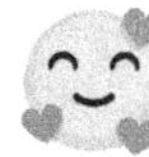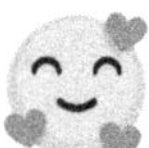

44. Split pea soup

Let's do that and fill in the time here Prep Time :   Cook Time :   Servings :

Is this dish easy or difficult for you to make?

 ○   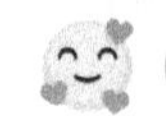 ○

Write 5 friends with whom you want to share this dish

....
....
....
....
....

INGREDIENTS

- 1 tablespoon olive oil
- 1 onion, diced
- 2 carrots, peeled and diced
- 2 celery stalks, diced
- 3 cloves garlic, minced
- 1 pound dried split peas, rinsed
- 6 cups low-sodium vegetable or chicken broth
- 1 bay leaf
- 1 teaspoon dried thyme
- Salt and black pepper to taste
- Chopped fresh parsley for garnish (optional)

1. In a large pot or Dutch oven, heat the olive oil over medium heat. Add the diced onion, carrots, and celery. Sauté for 5-7 minutes, until the vegetables are softened.

2. Add the minced garlic and sauté for an additional 1-2 minutes, until fragrant.

3. Stir in the rinsed split peas, broth, bay leaf, and dried thyme. Bring the mixture to a boil.

4. Reduce the heat to low, cover the pot, and let the soup simmer for 45-60 minutes, stirring occasionally, until the split peas are very soft and the soup has thickened.

5. Remove the bay leaf. Use an immersion blender or a regular blender to puree the soup to your desired consistency.

6. Season the split pea soup with salt and black pepper to taste.

7. Serve the soup hot, garnished with chopped fresh parsley (if desired).

This soup is a great way to incorporate the MIND diet principles:

- Split peas are a good source of protein, fiber, and folate, all of which are important for brain health.

- Vegetables like carrots, celery, and onions provide antioxidants and other beneficial compounds.

- Herbs like thyme have anti-inflammatory properties that may help protect the brain.

This soup is easy to prepare, comforting, and satisfying. It makes a great lunch or dinner option for seniors following the MIND diet.

How would you rate this dish?

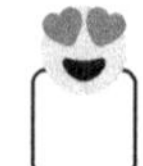 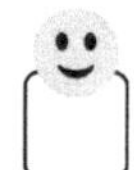 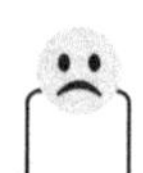 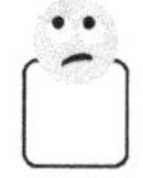 

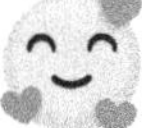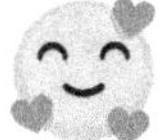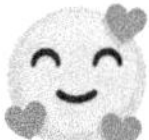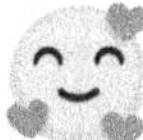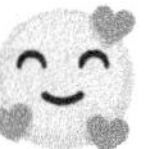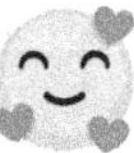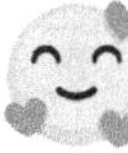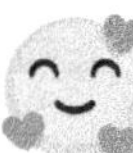

45. Chicken and vegetable soup

Is this dish easy or difficult for you to make?

Write 5 friends with whom you want to share this dish

....
....
....
....

INGREDIENTS

- 1 tablespoon olive oil
- 1 onion, diced
- 2 carrots, peeled and diced
- 2 celery stalks, diced
- 3 cloves garlic, minced
- 4 cups low-sodium chicken broth
- 2 cups shredded cooked chicken (about 1 lb)
- 1 cup frozen peas
- 1 cup chopped kale or spinach
- 1 bay leaf
- 1 teaspoon dried thyme
- Salt and black pepper to taste
- Chopped fresh parsley for garnish (optional)

1. In a large pot or Dutch oven, heat the olive oil over medium heat. Add the diced onion, carrots, and celery. Sauté for 5-7 minutes, until the vegetables are softened.

2. Add the minced garlic and sauté for an additional 1-2 minutes, until fragrant.

3. Pour in the chicken broth and add the shredded cooked chicken, frozen peas, chopped kale or spinach, bay leaf, and dried thyme.

4. Bring the soup to a simmer and let it cook for 15-20 minutes, allowing the flavors to meld.

5. Remove the bay leaf. Season the soup with salt and black pepper to taste.

6. Serve the chicken and vegetable soup hot, garnished with chopped fresh parsley (if desired).

This soup is a great way to incorporate the MIND diet principles:

- Chicken is a lean protein that is important for brain health and cognitive function.

- Vegetables like carrots, celery, kale, and peas are rich in antioxidants and other beneficial compounds.

- Herbs like thyme have anti-inflammatory properties that may help protect the brain.

This soup is easy to prepare, comforting, and satisfying. It makes a great lunch or dinner option for seniors following the MIND diet.

You can also add whole-grain crackers or a slice of whole-grain bread to make it a more complete meal.

How would you rate this dish?

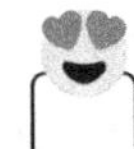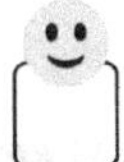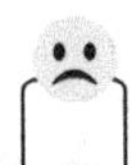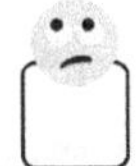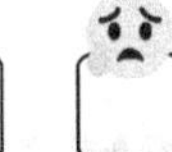

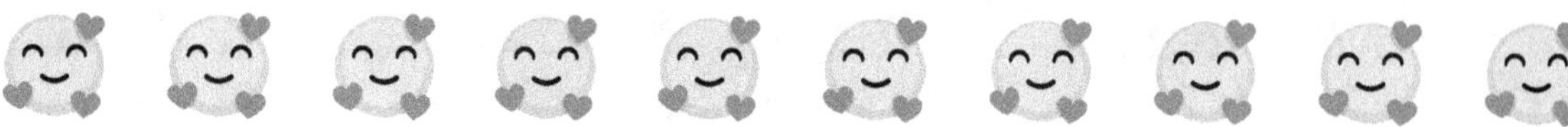

46. Mushroom barley soup

Let's do that and fill in the time here   Prep Time :   Cook Time :   Servings :

Is this dish easy or difficult for you to make?

 ◯   ◯

Write 5 friends with whom you want to share this dish

....

....

....

....

....

INGREDIENTS

- 2 tablespoons olive oil
- 1 onion, diced
- 8 ounces cremini or button mushrooms, sliced
- 3 cloves garlic, minced
- 1 cup pearl barley, rinsed
- 6 cups low-sodium vegetable or chicken broth
- 2 bay leaves
- 1 teaspoon dried thyme
- Salt and black pepper to taste
- Chopped fresh parsley for garnish (optional)

1. In a large pot or Dutch oven, heat the olive oil over medium heat. Add the diced onion and sauté for 5-7 minutes, until translucent.

2. Add the sliced mushrooms and sauté for an additional 5 minutes, until the mushrooms are softened.

3. Stir in the minced garlic and sauté for 1-2 minutes, until fragrant.

4. Pour in the rinsed pearl barley and the broth. Add the bay leaves and dried thyme.

5. Bring the soup to a boil, then reduce the heat to low, cover the pot, and let the soup simmer for 45-60 minutes, or until the barley is tender.

6. Remove the bay leaves. Season the soup with salt and black pepper to taste.

7. Serve the mushroom barley soup hot, garnished with chopped fresh parsley (if desired).

This soup is a great way to incorporate the MIND diet principles:

- Barley is a whole grain that provides fiber, protein, and other nutrients important for brain health.

- Mushrooms are a good source of antioxidants and anti-inflammatory compounds that may help protect the brain.

- Herbs like thyme have been shown to have neuroprotective effects.

This soup is easy to prepare, comforting, and satisfying. It makes a great lunch or dinner option for seniors following the MIND diet.

How would you rate this dish?

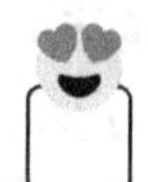  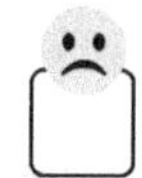 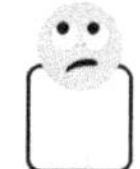 

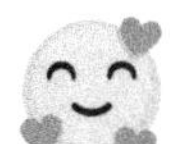 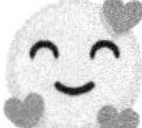 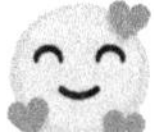 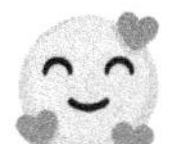 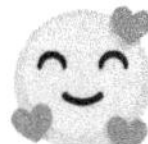 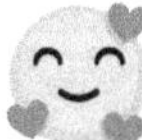 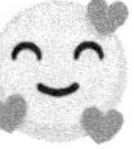 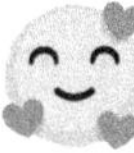 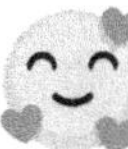 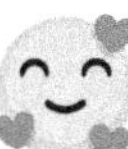

47. Carrot ginger soup

Is this dish easy or difficult for you to make?

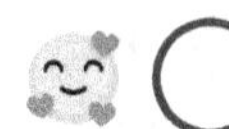

Write 5 friends with whom you want to share this dish

....
....
....
....

INGREDIENTS

- 2 tablespoons olive oil
- 1 onion, diced
- 3 cloves garlic, minced
- 1 tablespoon grated fresh ginger
- 1 pound carrots, peeled and sliced
- 4 cups low-sodium vegetable or chicken broth
- 1 cup unsweetened almond milk (or regular milk)
- 1 teaspoon ground cumin
- 1/4 teaspoon ground cinnamon
- Salt and black pepper to taste
- Chopped fresh parsley for garnish (optional)

1. In a large pot or Dutch oven, heat the olive oil over medium heat. Add the diced onion and sauté for 5-7 minutes, until translucent.

2. Add the minced garlic and grated ginger. Sauté for an additional 1-2 minutes, until fragrant.

3. Stir in the sliced carrots, broth, almond milk (or regular milk), ground cumin, and ground cinnamon.

4. Bring the soup to a simmer, then reduce the heat to low, cover the pot, and let the soup cook for 25-30 minutes, or until the carrots are very soft.

5. Using an immersion blender or a regular blender, puree the soup until smooth and creamy.

6. Season the carrot ginger soup with salt and black pepper to taste.

7. Serve the soup hot, garnished with chopped fresh parsley (if desired).

This soup is a great way to incorporate the MIND diet principles:

- Carrots are a rich source of beta-carotene, an antioxidant that has been linked to improved cognitive function.

- Ginger has anti-inflammatory properties that may help protect the brain.

- The almond milk (or regular milk) provides a creamy texture and a boost of protein.

This soup is easy to prepare, comforting, and satisfying. It makes a great lunch or dinner option for seniors following the MIND diet.

How would you rate this dish?

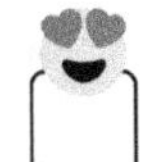 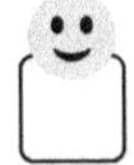 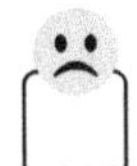 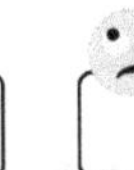 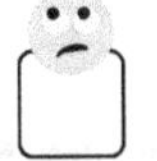 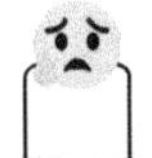

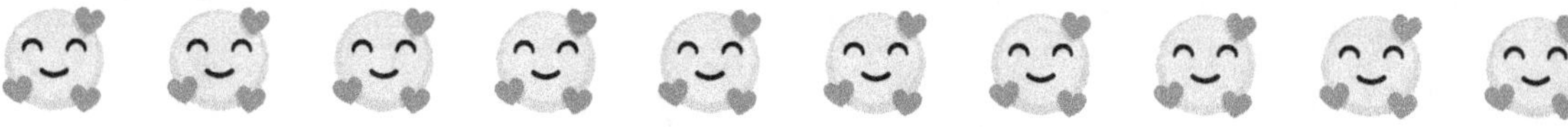

48. Broccoli and cheddar soup (light on cheese)

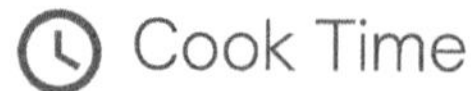 Prep Time :

 Cook Time :

Servings :

Is this dish easy or difficult for you to make?

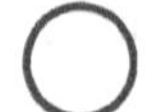 ◯   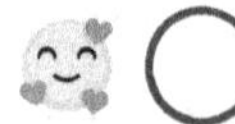 ◯

Write 5 friends with whom you want to share this dish

....
....
....
....
....

INGREDIENTS

- 2 tablespoons olive oil
- 1 onion, diced
- 3 cloves garlic, minced
- 4 cups chopped broccoli florets
- 3 cups low-sodium chicken or vegetable broth
- 1 cup unsweetened almond milk (or low-fat milk)
- 1/2 cup shredded low-fat cheddar cheese
- 1 teaspoon Dijon mustard
- 1/4 teaspoon ground nutmeg
- Salt and black pepper to taste
- Chopped fresh parsley for garnish (optional)

1. In a large pot or Dutch oven, heat the olive oil over medium heat. Add the diced onion and sauté for 5-7 minutes, until translucent.

2. Add the minced garlic and sauté for an additional 1-2 minutes, until fragrant.

3. Stir in the chopped broccoli florets and the broth. Bring the mixture to a simmer.

4. Reduce the heat to low, cover the pot, and let the broccoli cook for 15-20 minutes, or until very tender.

5. Using an immersion blender or a regular blender, puree the soup until smooth and creamy.

6. Return the pureed soup to the pot and stir in the almond milk (or low-fat milk), shredded cheddar cheese, Dijon mustard, and ground nutmeg.

7. Heat the soup over low heat, stirring occasionally, until the cheese is melted and the soup is heated through.

8. Season the broccoli and cheddar soup with salt and black pepper to taste.

9. Serve the soup hot, garnished with chopped fresh parsley (if desired).

This soup is a great way to incorporate the MIND diet principles:

- Broccoli is a cruciferous vegetable that is rich in antioxidants and other brain-boosting compounds.
- The reduced amount of cheddar cheese keeps the dish light and heart-healthy.
- Almond milk (or low-fat milk) provides a creamy texture without too much saturated fat

How would you rate this dish?

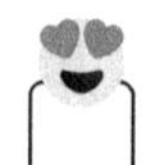 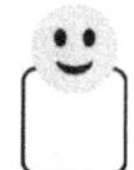 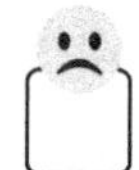 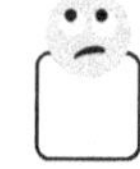 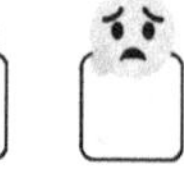

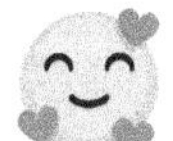 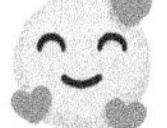 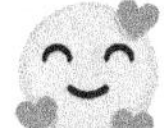 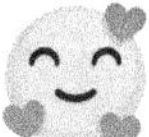 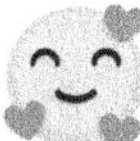 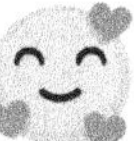 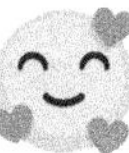 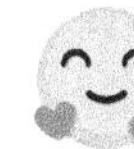  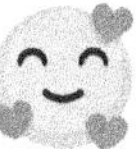 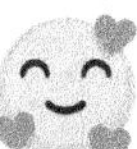

49. Sweet potato and black bean soup

Prep Time : Cook Time : Servings :

Is this dish easy or difficult for you to make?

Write 5 friends with whom you want to share this dish
....
....
....
....

INGREDIENTS

- 2 tablespoons olive oil
- 1 onion, diced
- 3 cloves garlic, minced
- 2 medium sweet potatoes, peeled and cubed
- 1 (15-ounce) can black beans, rinsed and drained
- 4 cups low-sodium vegetable or chicken broth
- 1 teaspoon ground cumin
- 1/2 teaspoon chili powder
- 1/4 teaspoon ground cinnamon
- Salt and black pepper to taste
- Chopped fresh cilantro for garnish (optional)

How would you rate this dish?

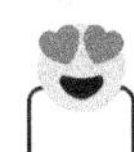 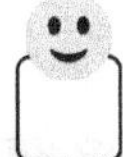 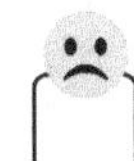 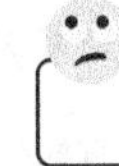 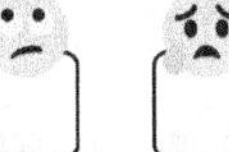

1. In a large pot or Dutch oven, heat the olive oil over medium heat. Add the diced onion and sauté for 5-7 minutes, until translucent.

2. Add the minced garlic and sauté for an additional 1-2 minutes, until fragrant.

3. Stir in the cubed sweet potatoes, rinsed and drained black beans, broth, ground cumin, chili powder, and ground cinnamon.

4. Bring the soup to a simmer, then reduce the heat to low, cover the pot, and let the soup cook for 25-30 minutes, or until the sweet potatoes are very soft.

5. Using an immersion blender or a regular blender, puree the soup until smooth and creamy.

6. Season the sweet potato and black bean soup with salt and black pepper to taste.

7. Serve the soup hot, garnished with chopped fresh cilantro (if desired).

This soup is a great way to incorporate the MIND diet principles:

- Sweet potatoes are a rich source of beta-carotene, an antioxidant that has been linked to improved cognitive function.
- Black beans are a good source of protein, fiber, and folate, all of which are important for brain health.
- Spices like cumin and cinnamon have anti-inflammatory properties that may help protect the brain.

This soup is easy to prepare, comforting, and satisfying. It makes a great lunch or dinner option for seniors following the MIND diet.

50. Red lentil soup

 Prep Time :   Cook Time :   Servings :

Is this dish easy or difficult for you to make?

 ◯   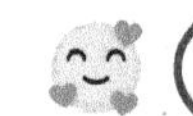 ◯

Write 5 ....
friends
with ....
whom
you ....
want to
share ....
this
dish ....

INGREDIENTS

- 2 tablespoons olive oil
- 1 onion, diced
- 3 cloves garlic, minced
- 1 tablespoon grated fresh ginger
- 1 cup red lentils, rinsed
- 6 cups low-sodium vegetable or chicken broth
- 1 teaspoon ground cumin
- 1/2 teaspoon ground coriander
- 1/4 teaspoon ground turmeric
- Salt and black pepper to taste
- Chopped fresh parsley or cilantro for garnish (optional)

How would you rate this dish?

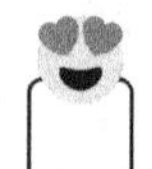  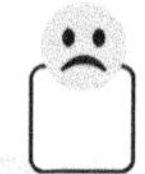 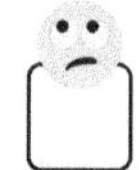 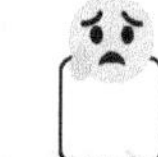

1. In a large pot or Dutch oven, heat the olive oil over medium heat. Add the diced onion and sauté for 5-7 minutes, until translucent.

2. Add the minced garlic and grated ginger. Sauté for an additional 1-2 minutes, until fragrant.

3. Stir in the rinsed red lentils, broth, ground cumin, ground coriander, and ground turmeric.

4. Bring the soup to a simmer, then reduce the heat to low, cover the pot, and let the soup cook for 20-25 minutes, or until the lentils are very soft.

5. Using an immersion blender or a regular blender, puree the soup until smooth and creamy.

6. Season the red lentil soup with salt and black pepper to taste.

7. Serve the soup hot, garnished with chopped fresh parsley or cilantro (if desired).

This soup is a great way to incorporate the MIND diet principles:

- Red lentils are a good source of protein, fiber, and folate, all of which are important for brain health.
- Ginger and turmeric have anti-inflammatory properties that may help protect the brain.
- The blend of spices, including cumin and coriander, adds flavor and additional brain-boosting benefits.

This soup is easy to prepare, comforting, and satisfying. It makes a great lunch or dinner option for seniors following the MIND diet.

You can also add diced carrots, celery, or other vegetables to boost the nutrient content even further.

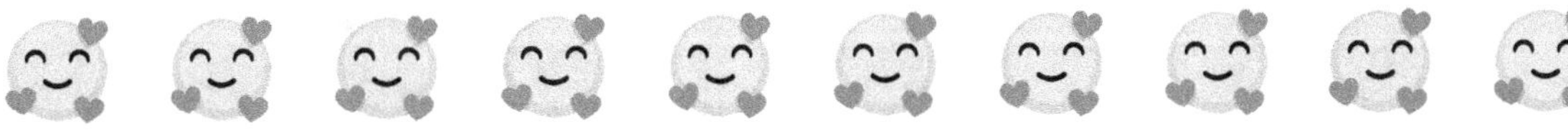

51. Kale and quinoa salad with a lemon vinaigrette

Let's do that and fill in the time here  Prep Time :   Cook Time :   Servings :

Is this dish easy or difficult for you to make?

○   ○

Write 5 friends with whom you want to share this dish ....

INGREDIENTS

For the salad:
- 4 cups chopped kale, stems removed
- 1 cup cooked quinoa, cooled
- 1/2 cup diced cucumber
- 1/4 cup diced red onion
- 1/4 cup toasted slivered almonds

For the lemon vinaigrette:
- 2 tablespoons olive oil
- 2 tablespoons freshly squeezed lemon juice
- 1 teaspoon Dijon mustard
- 1 teaspoon honey
- 1 clove garlic, minced
- Salt and black pepper to taste

1. In a large bowl, combine the chopped kale, cooked quinoa, diced cucumber, diced red onion, and toasted slivered almonds.

2. In a small bowl, whisk together the olive oil, lemon juice, Dijon mustard, honey, and minced garlic. Season the vinaigrette with salt and black pepper to taste.

3. Drizzle the lemon vinaigrette over the kale and quinoa salad and toss gently to coat.

4. Let the salad sit for 5-10 minutes to allow the flavors to meld. Serve the kale and quinoa salad chilled or at room temperature.

This salad is a great way to incorporate the MIND diet principles:

- Kale is a nutrient-dense leafy green that is rich in antioxidants and other brain-boosting compounds.

- Quinoa is a whole grain that provides complex carbohydrates, protein, and fiber, all of which are important for brain health.

- Almonds are a good source of healthy fats, vitamin E, and other nutrients that support cognitive function.

- The lemon vinaigrette provides a bright, tangy flavor and contains anti-inflammatory compounds.

This salad is easy to prepare, refreshing, and satisfying. It makes a great lunch or side dish option for seniors following the MIND diet.

You can also add other vegetables, such as diced bell peppers or cherry tomatoes, to further boost the nutrient content.

How would you rate this dish?

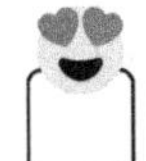 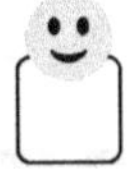 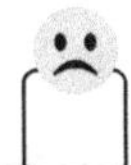 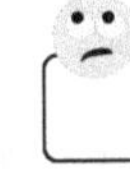 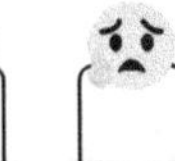

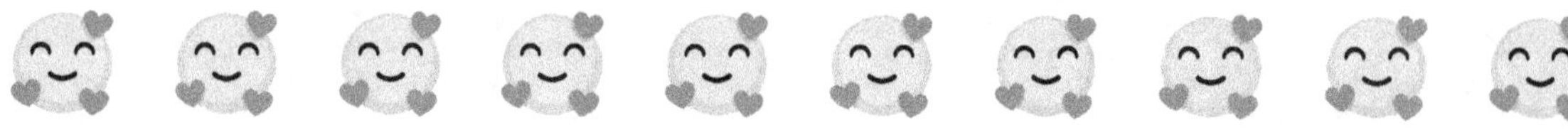

52. Spinach and strawberry salad with balsamic dressing

 Prep Time :   Cook Time :   Servings :

Is this dish easy or difficult for you to make?

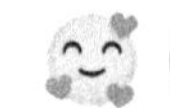 ◯   ◯

Write 5 friends with whom you want to share this dish ....

INGREDIENTS

For the salad:
- 5 cups fresh spinach leaves, washed and dried
- 1 cup fresh strawberries, sliced
- 1/4 cup toasted slivered almonds
- 2 tablespoons crumbled feta cheese (optional)

For the balsamic dressing:
- 2 tablespoons balsamic vinegar
- 1 tablespoon olive oil
- 1 teaspoon Dijon mustard
- 1 teaspoon honey
- 1 clove garlic, minced
- Salt and black pepper to taste

1. In a large salad bowl, combine the fresh spinach leaves, sliced strawberries, toasted slivered almonds, and crumbled feta cheese (if using).

2. In a small bowl, whisk together the balsamic vinegar, olive oil, Dijon mustard, honey, and minced garlic. Season the dressing with salt and black pepper to taste.

3. Drizzle the balsamic dressing over the spinach and strawberry salad and toss gently to coat.

4. Serve the salad immediately, or refrigerate until ready to serve.

This spinach and strawberry salad is a great option for a light and refreshing meal or side dish. It's packed with nutrients that support overall health, including:

- Spinach is a nutrient-dense leafy green that is rich in antioxidants, vitamins, and minerals.

- Strawberries are a good source of vitamin C, fiber, and antioxidants.

- Almonds provide healthy fats, protein, and vitamin E

- The balsamic dressing adds a tangy, sweet flavor and contains anti-inflammatory compounds.

This salad is easy to prepare and can be enjoyed year-round. It's a great way to incorporate fresh, seasonal produce into your diet.

Feel free to adjust the ingredient amounts to suit your preferences or the number of servings you need. Enjoy this delicious and nutritious spinach and strawberry salad!

How would you rate this dish?

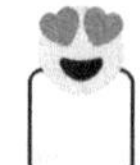 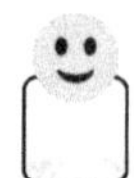  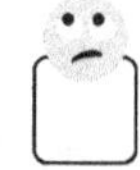 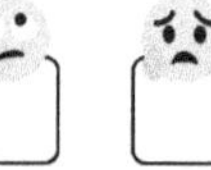

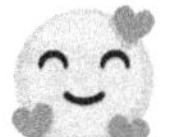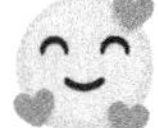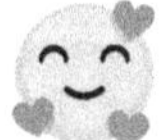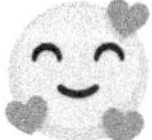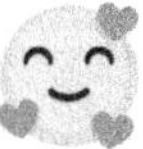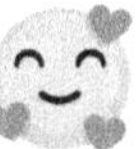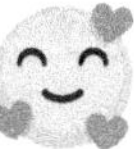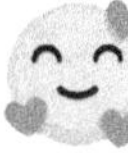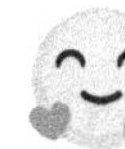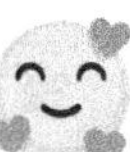

53. Arugula and beet salad with goat cheese

Let's do that and fill in the time here ✓ Prep Time :   🕐 Cook Time :   🍴 Servings :

Is this dish easy or difficult for you to make?

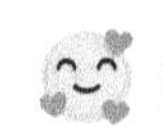 ◯   ◯

Write 5 ....
friends
with   ....
whom
you   ....
want to
share ....
this
dish   ....

INGREDIENTS

- 5 cups baby arugula
- 2 medium beets, roasted, peeled, and sliced
- 1/4 cup crumbled goat cheese
- 2 tablespoons toasted walnuts
- 2 tablespoons balsamic vinegar
- 1 tablespoon olive oil
- 1 teaspoon Dijon mustard
- 1 teaspoon honey
- Salt and black pepper to taste

How would you rate this dish?

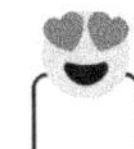 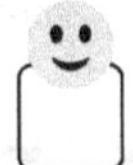 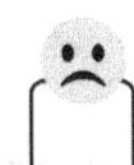 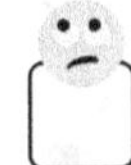 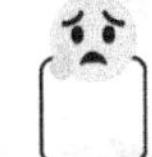

1. In a large salad bowl, combine the baby arugula, roasted and sliced beets, crumbled goat cheese, and toasted walnuts.

2. In a small bowl, whisk together the balsamic vinegar, olive oil, Dijon mustard, and honey. Season the dressing with salt and black pepper to taste.

3. Drizzle the balsamic dressing over the arugula and beet salad and toss gently to coat.

4. Serve the salad immediately, or refrigerate until ready to serve.

This arugula and beet salad is a great way to incorporate the MIND diet principles:

- Arugula is a nutrient-dense leafy green that is rich in antioxidants and other brain-boosting compounds.

- Beets are a good source of betalains, which have anti-inflammatory properties and may help protect the brain.

- Goat cheese provides a creamy texture and a boost of protein.

- Walnuts are a rich source of omega-3 fatty acids, which are important for cognitive function.

This salad is easy to prepare, refreshing, and satisfying. It makes a great lunch or side dish option for seniors following the MIND diet.

You can also add other vegetables, such as sliced cucumber or cherry tomatoes, to further boost the nutrient content.

Enjoy this delicious and nutritious arugula and beet salad with goat cheese!

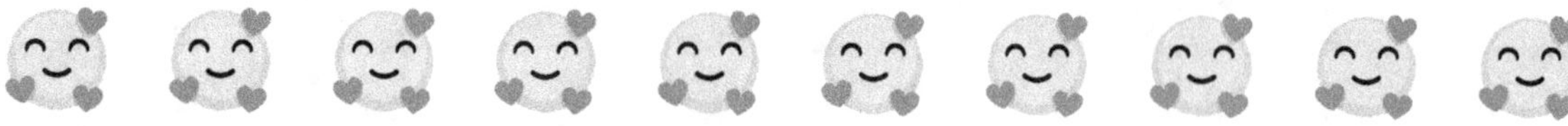

54. Chickpea and cucumber salad with dill dressing

Prep Time :   Cook Time :   Servings :

Is this dish easy or difficult for you to make?

 ◯   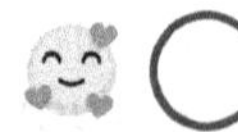 ◯

Write 5 friends with whom you want to share this dish

....

....

....

....

....

INGREDIENTS

For the salad:
- 1 (15-ounce) can chickpeas, rinsed and drained
- 1 cucumber, diced
- 1/2 red onion, thinly sliced
- 1/4 cup chopped fresh dill
- 2 tablespoons chopped fresh parsley

For the dill dressing:
- 1/4 cup plain Greek yogurt
- 2 tablespoons olive oil
- 2 tablespoons white wine vinegar
- 1 tablespoon chopped fresh dill
- 1 clove garlic, minced
- Salt and black pepper to taste

How would you rate this dish?

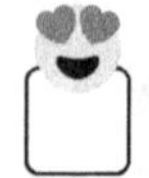 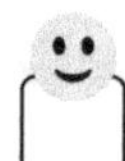 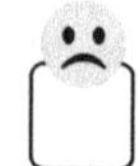 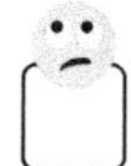 

1. In a large bowl, combine the rinsed and drained chickpeas, diced cucumber, thinly sliced red onion, chopped fresh dill, and chopped fresh parsley.

2. In a small bowl, whisk together the Greek yogurt, olive oil, white wine vinegar, chopped fresh dill, and minced garlic. Season the dressing with salt and black pepper to taste.

3. Drizzle the dill dressing over the chickpea and cucumber salad and toss gently to coat.

4. Refrigerate the salad for at least 30 minutes to allow the flavors to meld.

5. Serve the chickpea and cucumber salad chilled or at room temperature.

This salad is a great way to incorporate the MIND diet principles:

- Chickpeas are a good source of protein, fiber, and folate, all of which are important for brain health.

- Cucumbers are hydrating and contain antioxidants that may help protect the brain.

- Dill is an herb with anti-inflammatory properties that may benefit cognitive function.

- The Greek yogurt in the dressing provides a creamy texture and a boost of protein.

This salad is easy to prepare, refreshing, and satisfying. It makes a great lunch or side dish option for seniors following the MIND diet.

You can also add other vegetables, such as cherry tomatoes or bell peppers, to further boost the nutrient content.

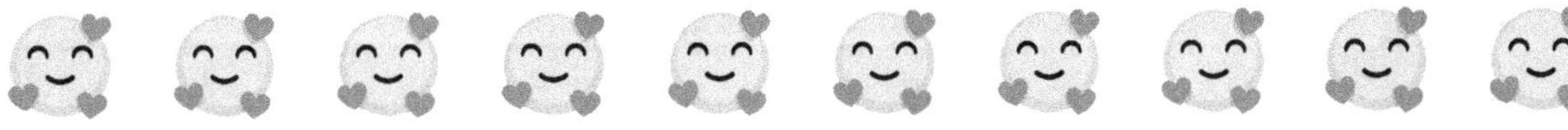

55. Mediterranean salad with olives, cucumbers, and feta

 *Let's do that and fill in the time here* (✓) Prep Time :   (◷) Cook Time :   Servings :

Is this dish easy or difficult for you to make?

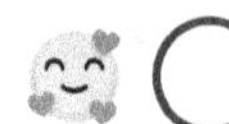 ○   ○

Write 5 ....
friends
with   ....
whom
you   ....
want to
share   ....
this
dish   ....

INGREDIENTS

- 5 cups mixed greens (such as spinach, arugula, or romaine)
- 1 cucumber, diced
- 1/2 cup pitted kalamata olives, halved
- 1/4 cup crumbled feta cheese
- 1/4 cup chopped fresh parsley
- 2 tablespoons olive oil
- 2 tablespoons red wine vinegar
- 1 teaspoon Dijon mustard
- 1 clove garlic, minced
- Salt and black pepper to taste

How would you rate this dish?

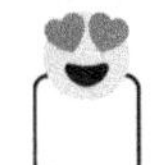 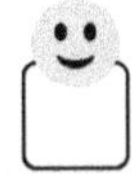 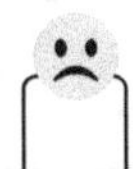 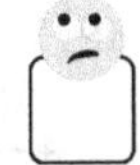 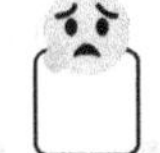

1. In a large salad bowl, combine the mixed greens, diced cucumber, halved kalamata olives, crumbled feta cheese, and chopped fresh parsley.

2. In a small bowl, whisk together the olive oil, red wine vinegar, Dijon mustard, and minced garlic. Season the dressing with salt and black pepper to taste.

3. Drizzle the Mediterranean dressing over the salad and toss gently to coat. Serve the salad immediately, or refrigerate until ready to serve.

This Mediterranean salad is a great way to incorporate the MIND diet principles:

- Mixed greens, such as spinach and arugula, are nutrient-dense and rich in antioxidants.

- Cucumbers are hydrating and contain compounds that may help protect the brain.

- Kalamata olives are a good source of healthy monounsaturated fats and antioxidants.

- Feta cheese provides a boost of protein and calcium.

- The Mediterranean dressing contains olive oil, which is a key component of the MIND diet.

This salad is easy to prepare, refreshing, and satisfying. It makes a great lunch or side dish option for seniors following the MIND diet.

You can also add other Mediterranean-inspired ingredients, such as cherry tomatoes, roasted red peppers, or grilled chicken, to make it a more substantial meal.

Enjoy this delicious and nutritious Mediterranean salad!

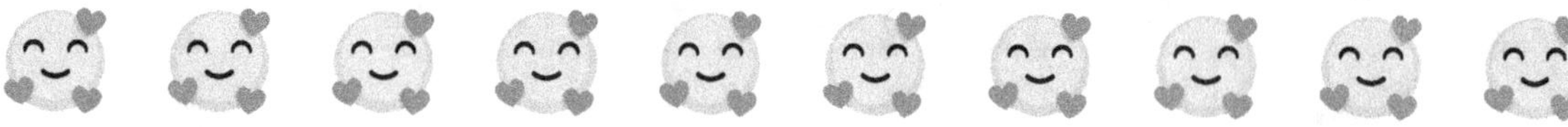

56. Roasted vegetable salad with balsamic glaze

Let's do that and fill in the time here  Prep Time :   Cook Time :   Servings :

Is this dish easy or difficult for you to make?

○   ○

Write 5 friends with whom you want to share this dish ....

INGREDIENTS

For the roasted vegetables:
- 2 cups cubed butternut squash
- 1 cup Brussels sprouts, halved
- 1 red bell pepper, diced
- 1 zucchini, diced
- 2 tablespoons olive oil
- Salt and black pepper to taste

For the salad:
- 5 cups mixed greens (such as spinach, arugula, or kale)
- 1/4 cup toasted walnuts
- 2 tablespoons crumbled feta cheese (optional)

For the balsamic glaze:
- 1/4 cup balsamic vinegar
- 1 tablespoon honey

How would you rate this dish?

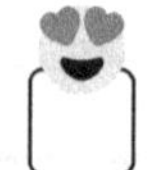 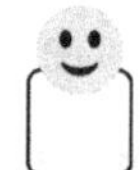 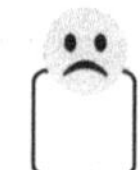 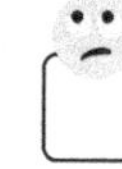 

1. Preheat your oven to 400°F (200°C).

2. In a large bowl, toss the cubed butternut squash, halved Brussels sprouts, diced red bell pepper, and diced zucchini with 2 tablespoons of olive oil. Season with salt and black pepper.

3. Spread the seasoned vegetables out on a baking sheet and roast in the preheated oven for 20-25 minutes, or until the vegetables are tender and lightly caramelized.

4. While the vegetables are roasting, make the balsamic glaze. In a small saucepan, combine the balsamic vinegar and honey. Bring the mixture to a simmer over medium heat and cook for 5-7 minutes, or until the glaze has thickened slightly.

5. In a large salad bowl, combine the mixed greens, roasted vegetables, toasted walnuts, and crumbled feta cheese (if using).

6. Drizzle the balsamic glaze over the salad and toss gently to coat. Serve the roasted vegetable salad immediately.

This salad is a great way to incorporate the MIND diet principles:

- The roasted vegetables, such as butternut squash and Brussels sprouts, are rich in antioxidants and other brain-boosting compounds.
- Walnuts provide a good source of omega-3 fatty acids, which are important for cognitive function.
- The balsamic glaze adds a sweet and tangy flavor, as well as anti-inflammatory properties.

This salad is easy to prepare, visually appealing, and satisfying. It makes a great lunch or side dish option for seniors following the MIND diet.

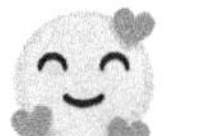 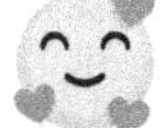 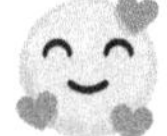 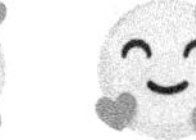 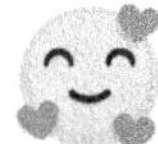 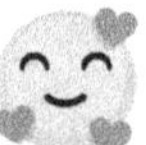 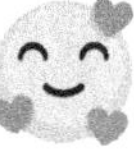 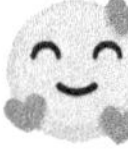 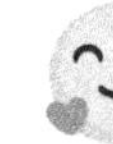 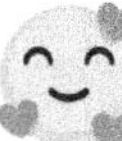

57. Waldorf salad with walnuts and apples

Prep Time :   Cook Time :   Servings :

Is this dish easy or difficult for you to make?

Write 5 friends with whom you want to share this dish

....

....

....

....

....

INGREDIENTS

- 3 medium apples, cored and chopped
- 1 cup chopped celery
- 1/2 cup chopped walnuts
- 1/2 cup mayonnaise
- 2 tablespoons lemon juice
- 1 tablespoon white sugar
- 1/4 teaspoon salt

1. In a large bowl, combine the chopped apples, celery, and walnuts.

2. In a small bowl, whisk together the mayonnaise, lemon juice, sugar, and salt until well combined.

3. Pour the dressing over the apple mixture and stir gently until everything is evenly coated.

4. Refrigerate the salad for at least 30 minutes before serving to allow the flavors to meld.

5. Serve chilled. This salad can be made a day in advance.

The classic Waldorf salad features apples, celery, and walnuts in a creamy dressing. The lemon juice helps prevent the apples from browning. This makes a refreshing side dish or light main course salad. Enjoy!

How would you rate this dish?

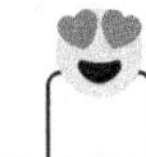 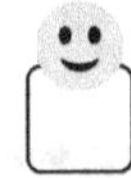  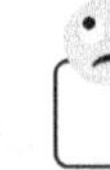 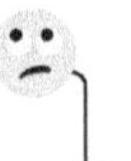 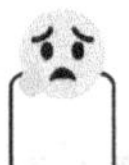

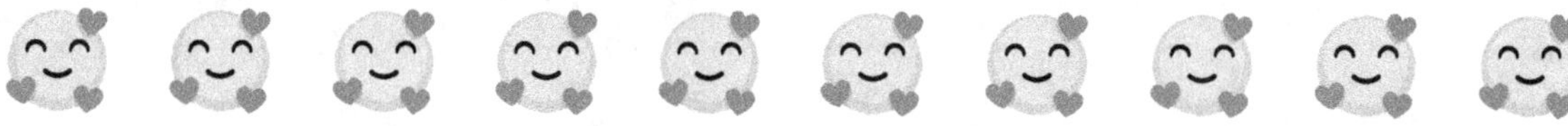

58. Farro salad with cherry tomatoes and basil

 Prep Time : Cook Time : Servings :

Is this dish easy or difficult for you to make?

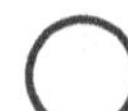 ◯ 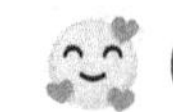 ◯

Write 5 friends with whom you want to share this dish

....

....

....

....

....

INGREDIENTS

- 1 cup dry farro, cooked according to package

1. In a large bowl, combine the cooked and cooled farro, cherry tomatoes, basil, and walnuts.

2. In a small bowl, whisk together the olive oil, balsamic vinegar, garlic, salt, and pepper.

3. Pour the dressing over the farro salad and toss gently to coat everything evenly.

4. Refrigerate for at least 30 minutes to allow the flavors to meld.

5. Serve chilled or at room temperature.

This salad is perfect for the MIND diet, which emphasizes foods that are good for brain health, such as whole grains (farro), vegetables (tomatoes), herbs (basil), and nuts (walnuts). The healthy fats, antioxidants, and fiber in this dish make it a nutritious and delicious option for seniors looking to support cognitive function.

How would you rate this dish?

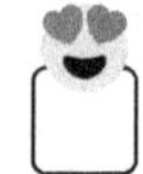 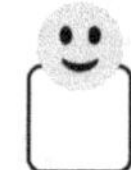 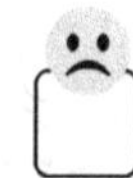 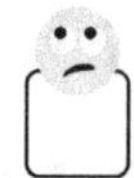  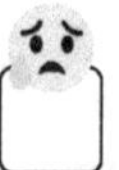

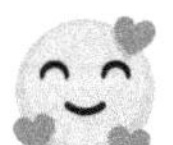 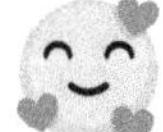 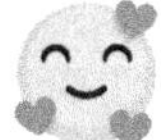 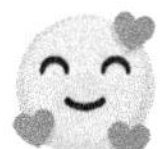 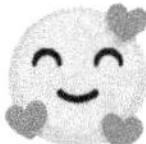 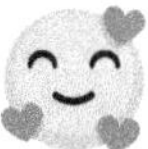 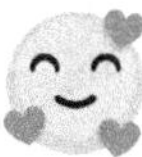 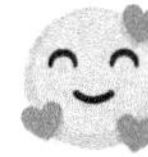 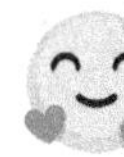 

59. Orzo salad with grilled zucchini and feta

Let's do that and fill in the time here Prep Time :   Cook Time :   Servings :

Is this dish easy or difficult for you to make?

Write 5 friends with whom you want to share this dish

....
....
....
....

INGREDIENTS

- 1 cup dry orzo pasta, cooked according to package

1. Preheat grill or grill pan to medium-high heat.

2. Brush the zucchini slices with 1 tablespoon of the olive oil and season with a pinch of salt and pepper.

3. Grill the zucchini for 2-3 minutes per side, until tender and lightly charred. Remove from grill and let cool slightly, then chop into bite-sized pieces.

4. In a large bowl, combine the cooked and cooled orzo, grilled zucchini, feta, basil, lemon juice, garlic, salt, and pepper. Drizzle with the remaining 1 tablespoon of olive oil and toss gently to coat.

5. Refrigerate the salad for at least 30 minutes to allow the flavors to meld.

6. Serve chilled or at room temperature.

This orzo salad is a great option for the MIND diet, which emphasizes whole grains (orzo), vegetables (zucchini), herbs (basil), and healthy fats (olive oil). The feta cheese also provides a boost of protein. This refreshing and flavorful dish is perfect for seniors looking to support brain health.

How would you rate this dish?

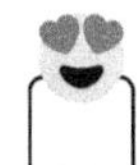 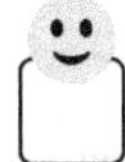 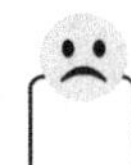 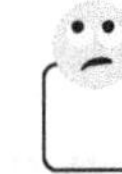 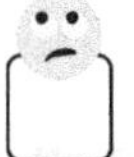 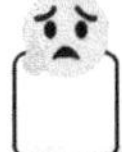

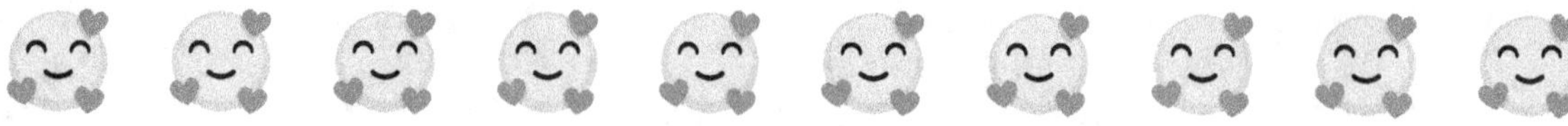

60. Mixed greens with mandarin oranges and almonds

Let's do that and fill in the time here ✓ Prep Time : 🕐 Cook Time : 🍴 Servings :

Is this dish easy or difficult for you to make?

 ◯   😊 ◯

Write 5 friends with whom you want to share this dish

....

....

....

....

....

INGREDIENTS

- 5 oz mixed greens (such as spinach, arugula, and kale)
- 1 (11 oz) can mandarin oranges, drained
- 1/4 cup sliced almonds, toasted
- 2 tablespoons balsamic vinegar
- 1 tablespoon extra-virgin olive oil
- 1 teaspoon Dijon mustard
- 1 teaspoon honey
- 1/4 teaspoon salt
- 1/4 teaspoon black pepper

1. In a large salad bowl, combine the mixed greens, mandarin oranges, and toasted almonds.

2. In a small bowl, whisk together the balsamic vinegar, olive oil, Dijon mustard, honey, salt, and pepper until well combined.

3. Drizzle the dressing over the salad and toss gently to coat.

4. Serve immediately.

This salad is a great option for the MIND diet, which emphasizes leafy green vegetables, berries, nuts, and healthy fats. The mandarin oranges provide a sweet citrus flavor, while the almonds add a satisfying crunch. The balsamic vinaigrette dressing is light and flavorful, complementing the other ingredients perfectly.

This refreshing and nutrient-dense salad is an excellent choice for seniors looking to support brain health and cognitive function through their diet.

How would you rate this dish?

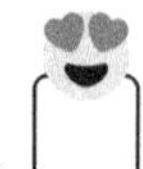 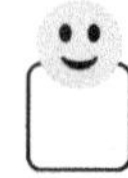   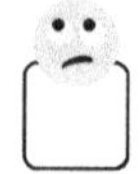 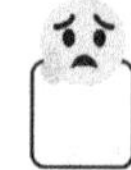

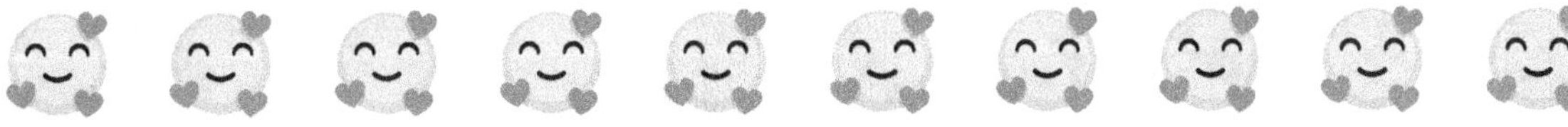

61. Stuffed zucchini boats with quinoa and vegetables

Prep Time :   Cook Time :   Servings :

Is this dish easy or difficult for you to make?

 ◯   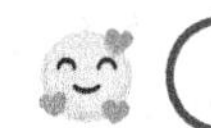 ◯

Write 5 friends with whom you want to share this dish

....

....

....

....

....

INGREDIENTS

- 4 medium zucchini, halved lengthwise
- 1 cup cooked quinoa
- 1 cup diced tomatoes
- 1/2 cup diced bell pepper
- 1/2 cup diced onion
- 2 cloves garlic, minced
- 1/4 cup crumbled feta cheese
- 2 tablespoons chopped fresh basil
- 1 tablespoon olive oil
- 1/4 teaspoon salt
- 1/4 teaspoon black pepper

1. Preheat oven to 400°F. Scoop out the flesh from the zucchini halves, leaving a 1/4-inch shell. Finely chop the scooped-out zucchini flesh.

2. In a skillet, heat the olive oil over medium heat. Add the chopped zucchini flesh, diced bell pepper, onion, and garlic. Sauté for 5-7 minutes, until vegetables are tender.

3. Remove the skillet from heat and stir in the cooked quinoa, diced tomatoes, feta cheese, and fresh basil. Season with salt and pepper.

4. Spoon the quinoa mixture evenly into the zucchini boats, packing it in gently.

5. Place the stuffed zucchini boats on a baking sheet and bake for 20-25 minutes, until the zucchini is tender.

6. Serve the stuffed zucchini boats warm.

This dish is an excellent choice for the MIND diet, as it features vegetables (zucchini, bell pepper, tomatoes), whole grains (quinoa), and healthy fats (olive oil, feta cheese). The combination of nutrients supports brain health and cognitive function, making it a great option for seniors over 60.

How would you rate this dish?

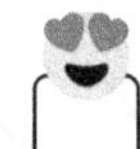 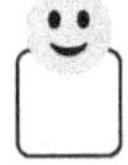 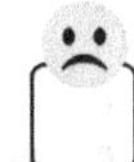 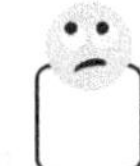 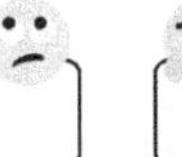 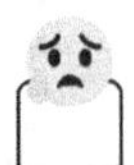

62. Black bean and corn tacos

 Prep Time :   Cook Time :   Servings :

Is this dish easy or difficult for you to make?

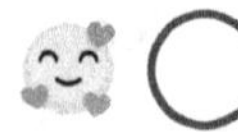 ◯   ◯

Write 5 ....
friends
with ....
whom
you ....
want to
share ....
this
dish ....

INGREDIENTS

- 1 (15 oz) can black beans, rinsed and drained
- 1 cup frozen corn kernels, thawed
- 1/2 cup diced onion
- 2 cloves garlic, minced
- 1 teaspoon ground cumin
- 1/2 teaspoon chili powder
- 1/4 teaspoon salt
- 8-10 small corn tortillas
- 1/2 cup shredded cabbage or lettuce
- 1/4 cup crumbled feta or queso fresco cheese
- 2 tablespoons chopped fresh cilantro
- 1 lime, cut into wedges

1. In a medium skillet, sauté the onion and garlic in a small amount of olive oil over medium heat for 2-3 minutes, until fragrant.

2. Add the black beans, corn, cumin, chili powder, and salt. Stir to combine and cook for 5-7 minutes, until heated through.

3. Warm the corn tortillas according to package instructions.

4. To assemble the tacos, place a spoonful of the black bean and corn mixture into each tortilla. Top with shredded cabbage or lettuce, crumbled feta or queso fresco, and chopped cilantro.

5. Serve the tacos with lime wedges for squeezing over the top.

This taco recipe is an excellent choice for the MIND diet, as it features whole grains (corn tortillas), legumes (black beans), vegetables (onion, cabbage/lettuce, cilantro), and healthy fats (feta/queso fresco). The combination of nutrients supports brain health and cognitive function, making it a great option for seniors over 60.

How would you rate this dish?

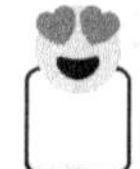 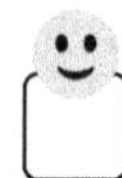 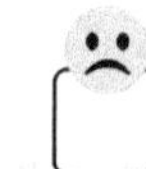 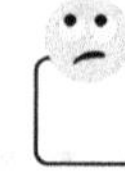 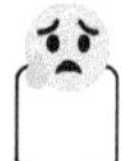

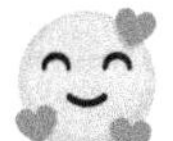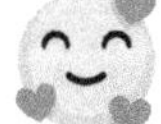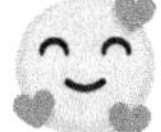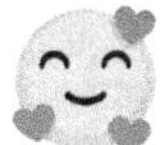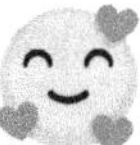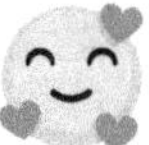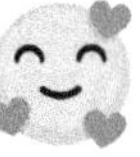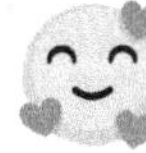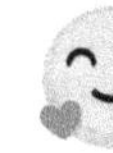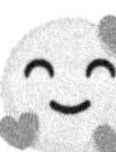

63. Spaghetti squash with marinara sauce

Let's do that and fill in the time here 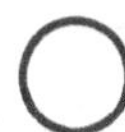 Prep Time :   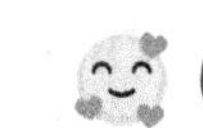 Cook Time :   Servings :

Is this dish easy or difficult for you to make?

Write 5 friends with whom you want to share this dish
....
....
....
....
....

INGREDIENTS

- 1 medium spaghetti squash, halved lengthwise and seeds removed
- 1 tablespoon olive oil
- 1/2 teaspoon salt
- 1/4 teaspoon black pepper
- 1 (24 oz) jar marinara sauce
- 1/4 cup grated Parmesan cheese (optional)
- 2 tablespoons chopped fresh basil (optional)

1. Preheat oven to 400°F. Line a baking sheet with parchment paper.

2. Place the spaghetti squash halves cut-side up on the prepared baking sheet. Drizzle with the olive oil and season with salt and pepper.

3. Roast the spaghetti squash for 40-50 minutes, until tender when pierced with a fork.

4. Remove the spaghetti squash from the oven and let cool slightly. Using a fork, gently scrape the flesh of the squash to create long, spaghetti-like strands.

5. In a large bowl, combine the spaghetti squash strands with the marinara sauce. Toss gently to coat.

6. Serve the spaghetti squash and marinara warm, topped with grated Parmesan cheese and chopped fresh basil, if desired.

This dish is an excellent choice for the MIND diet, as it features vegetables (spaghetti squash), healthy fats (olive oil), and antioxidants (from the marinara sauce). The combination of nutrients supports brain health and cognitive function, making it a great option for seniors over 60.

How would you rate this dish?

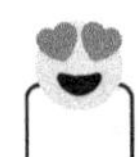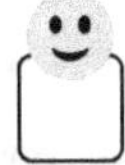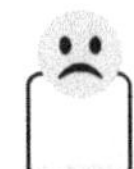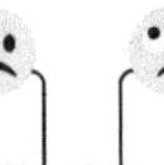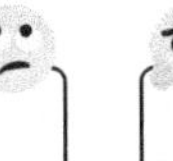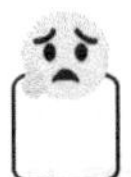

64. Vegetable stir-fry with tofu

Let's do that and fill in the time here  Prep Time :   Cook Time :   Servings :

Is this dish easy or difficult for you to make?

😭 ○   🥰 ○

Write 5 friends with whom you want to share this dish ....

INGREDIENTS

- 1 block (14 oz) extra-firm tofu, drained and cubed
- 2 tablespoons sesame oil, divided
- 2 cups broccoli florets
- 1 cup sliced mushrooms
- 1 red bell pepper, sliced
- 1 cup snow peas or snap peas
- 3 cloves garlic, minced
- 1 tablespoon grated fresh ginger
- 2 tablespoons low-sodium soy sauce
- 1 tablespoon rice vinegar
- 1 teaspoon honey
- 1/4 teaspoon red pepper flakes (optional)
- 2 cups cooked brown rice, for serving

1. In a large skillet or wok, heat 1 tablespoon of the sesame oil over medium-high heat. Add the cubed tofu and cook, stirring occasionally, until lightly browned on all sides, about 5-7 minutes. Transfer the tofu to a plate and set aside.

2. In the same skillet, heat the remaining 1 tablespoon of sesame oil over medium-high heat. Add the broccoli, mushrooms, bell pepper, and snow peas. Stir-fry for 3-4 minutes, until the vegetables are crisp-tender.

3. Add the garlic and ginger to the skillet and cook for 1 minute, until fragrant.

4. In a small bowl, whisk together the soy sauce, rice vinegar, honey, and red pepper flakes (if using).

5. Add the cooked tofu back to the skillet and pour the soy sauce mixture over the top. Toss everything together and cook for 2-3 minutes, until the sauce has thickened slightly.

6. Serve the vegetable stir-fry immediately over the cooked brown rice.

This stir-fry is a great vegetarian option that is packed with nutrient-dense vegetables and protein-rich tofu. The combination of flavors and textures makes it a delicious and satisfying meal.

How would you rate this dish?

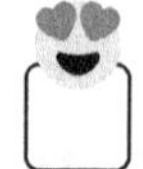 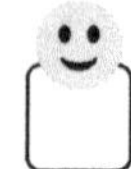 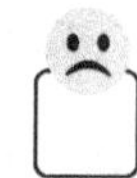 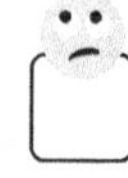 

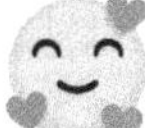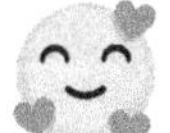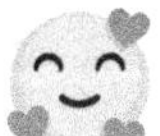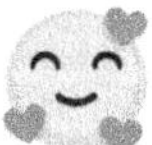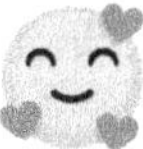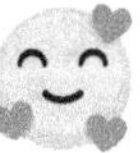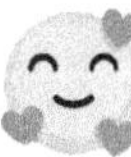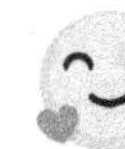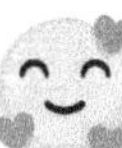

65. Lentil shepherd's pie

Let's do that and fill in the time here  Prep Time :   Cook Time :   Servings :

Is this dish easy or difficult for you to make?

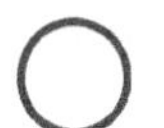 ◯    ◯

Write 5 friends with whom you want to share this dish

....

....

....

....

....

INGREDIENTS

For the Filling:
- 1 cup dry brown or green lentils, rinsed
- 3 cups vegetable broth
- 1 tablespoon olive oil
- 1 onion, diced
- 3 carrots, peeled and diced
- 3 celery stalks, diced
- 3 cloves garlic, minced
- 1 teaspoon dried thyme
- 1 teaspoon dried rosemary
- 1/2 teaspoon salt
- 1/4 teaspoon black pepper

For the Topping:
- 2 lbs Yukon Gold potatoes, peeled and cut into 1-inch cubes
- 1/4 cup unsweetened almond milk
- 2 tablespoons olive oil
- 1/2 teaspoon salt
- 1/4 teaspoon black pepper

How would you rate this dish?

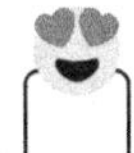 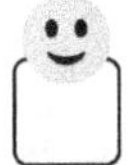 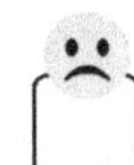 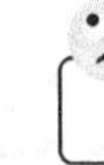 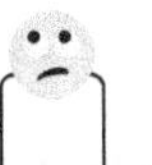 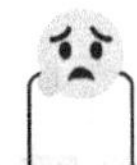

1. Preheat oven to 375°F.

2. In a medium saucepan, combine the lentils and vegetable broth. Bring to a boil, then reduce heat and simmer for 20-25 minutes, until lentils are tender. Drain any excess liquid and set aside.

3. In a large skillet, heat the olive oil over medium heat. Add the onion, carrots, celery, and garlic. Sauté for 5-7 minutes, until vegetables are softened.

4. Stir in the cooked lentils, thyme, rosemary, salt, and pepper. Cook for 2-3 minutes to blend the flavors.

5. Transfer the lentil mixture to a 9x13-inch baking dish.

6. In a large pot, cover the potato cubes with water and bring to a boil. Reduce heat and simmer for 15-20 minutes, until potatoes are tender. Drain and return to the pot.

7. Add the almond milk, olive oil, salt, and pepper to the potatoes. Mash until smooth and creamy.

8. Spread the mashed potatoes evenly over the lentil filling.

9. Bake for 25-30 minutes, until the potatoes are lightly browned.

10. Let cool for 5 minutes before serving.

This lentil shepherd's pie is a great MIND diet-friendly option, as it features legumes (lentils), vegetables (carrots, celery, potatoes), and healthy fats (olive oil). The combination of nutrients supports brain health and cognitive function, making it a great choice for seniors over 60.

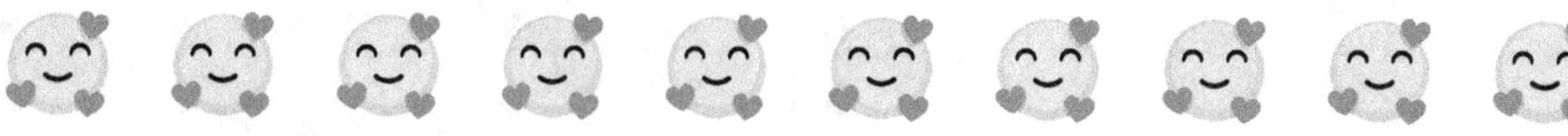

66. Grilled portobello mushrooms with garlic

Prep Time :   Cook Time :   Servings :

Is this dish easy or difficult for you to make?

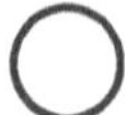 ◯    ◯

Write 5 friends with whom you want to share this dish

....

....

....

....

....

INGREDIENTS

- 4 large portobello mushroom caps, stems removed
- 2 tablespoons olive oil
- 3 cloves garlic, minced
- 1 teaspoon dried thyme
- 1/2 teaspoon salt
- 1/4 teaspoon black pepper

1. Preheat grill or grill pan to medium-high heat.

2. In a small bowl, whisk together the olive oil, minced garlic, dried thyme, salt, and black pepper.

3. Brush the mushroom caps all over with the garlic-herb oil, making sure to coat the tops and undersides.

4. Place the mushroom caps, gill-side up, directly on the grill grates. Grill for 4-5 minutes per side, until tender and lightly charred.

5. Transfer the grilled mushrooms to a serving platter.

6. Serve the portobello mushrooms warm, drizzling any remaining garlic-herb oil over the top.

These grilled portobello mushrooms make a delicious and easy side dish or vegetarian main course. The garlic and thyme add wonderful flavor, while grilling gives the mushrooms a nice smoky char.

Portobello mushrooms are an excellent source of antioxidants, vitamins, and minerals, making this a nutritious and MIND diet-friendly option. Enjoy these flavorful grilled mushrooms as part of a balanced meal.

How would you rate this dish?

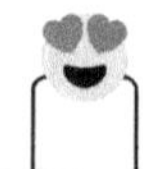 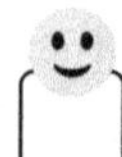 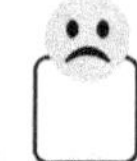 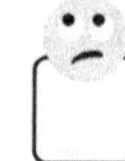 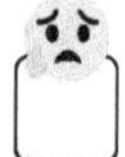

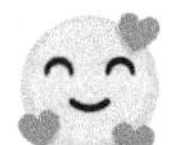 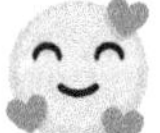 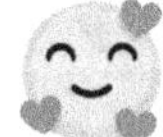 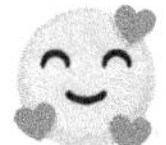 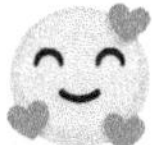 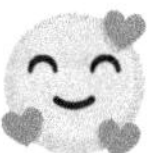 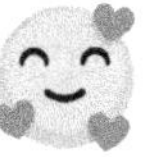 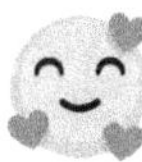 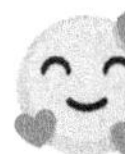 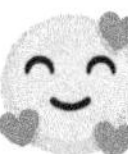

67. Chickpea and vegetable tagine

Prep Time :   **Cook Time :**   **Servings :**

Is this dish easy or difficult for you to make?

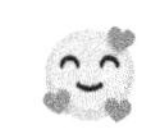 ◯   ◯

Write 5 friends with whom you want to share this dish

....
....
....
....

INGREDIENTS

- 2 tablespoons olive oil
- 1 onion, diced
- 3 cloves garlic, minced
- 1 teaspoon ground cumin
- 1 teaspoon ground coriander
- 1 teaspoon paprika
- 1/2 teaspoon ground cinnamon
- 1/4 teaspoon cayenne pepper (optional)
- 1 (15 oz) can chickpeas, drained and rinsed
- 1 (14 oz) can diced tomatoes
- 2 cups vegetable broth
- 2 medium carrots, peeled and sliced
- 1 medium zucchini, diced
- 1 cup cauliflower florets
- 1/4 cup chopped fresh parsley
- 1/4 cup chopped fresh cilantro
- Salt and black pepper to taste
- Cooked whole grain couscous or quinoa, for serving

1. In a large pot or Dutch oven, heat the olive oil over medium heat. Add the onion and sauté for 3-4 minutes until translucent.

2. Stir in the garlic, cumin, coriander, paprika, cinnamon, and cayenne (if using). Cook for 1 minute, until fragrant.

3. Add the chickpeas, diced tomatoes, vegetable broth, carrots, zucchini, and cauliflower. Bring the mixture to a simmer.

4. Reduce heat to medium-low and let the tagine simmer for 20-25 minutes, until the vegetables are tender.

5. Stir in the chopped parsley and cilantro. Season with salt and black pepper to taste.

6. Serve the chickpea and vegetable tagine warm, over a bed of cooked whole grain couscous or quinoa.

This tagine is an excellent choice for the MIND diet, as it features legumes (chickpeas), vegetables (carrots, zucchini, cauliflower), and herbs (parsley, cilantro). The combination of nutrients supports brain health and cognitive function, making it a great option for seniors over 60.

How would you rate this dish?

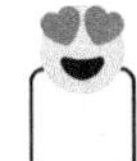 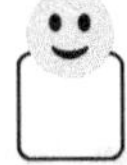 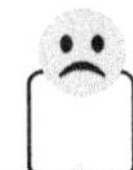 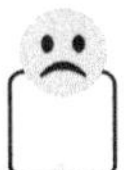 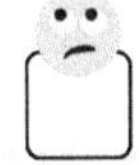 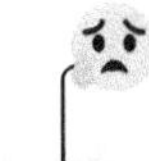 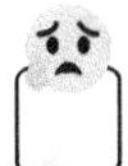

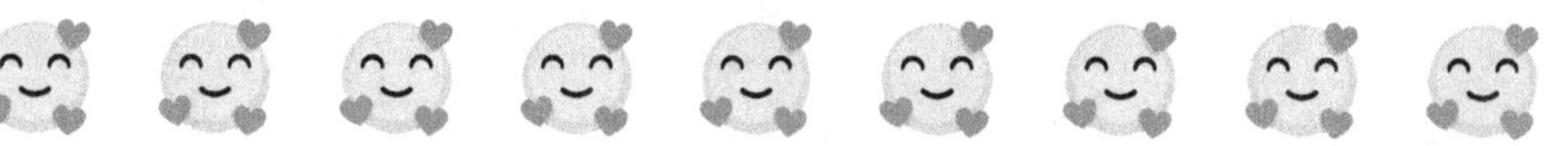

68. Cauliflower rice with peas and carrots

  Prep Time :   Cook Time :   Servings :

Is this dish easy or difficult for you to make?

 ◯   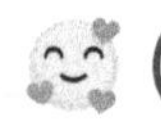 ◯

Write 5 ....
friends
with   ....
whom
you   ....
want to
share ....
this
dish   ....

INGREDIENTS

- 1 medium head of cauliflower, cut into florets
- 1 tablespoon olive oil
- 1 cup frozen peas
- 1 cup diced carrots
- 2 cloves garlic, minced
- 1/4 cup chopped fresh parsley
- 1/4 teaspoon salt
- 1/4 teaspoon black pepper

1. In a food processor, pulse the cauliflower florets in batches until they resemble the size and texture of rice. Set aside.

2. In a large skillet, heat the olive oil over medium heat. Add the diced carrots and sauté for 3-4 minutes, until they start to soften.

3. Add the frozen peas and minced garlic to the skillet. Cook for 1-2 minutes, until the garlic is fragrant.

4. Add the riced cauliflower to the skillet and stir to combine. Cook for 5-7 minutes, stirring occasionally, until the cauliflower is tender.

5. Remove the skillet from heat and stir in the chopped parsley, salt, and black pepper.

6. Serve the cauliflower rice with peas and carrots warm.

This cauliflower rice dish is an excellent choice for the MIND diet, as it features vegetables (cauliflower, carrots, peas) and herbs (parsley). The combination of nutrients supports brain health and cognitive function, making it a great option for seniors over 60.

Cauliflower is a cruciferous vegetable that is rich in antioxidants, while the peas and carrots provide additional vitamins and minerals. This simple, flavorful dish is a nutritious and delicious way to incorporate more MIND diet-friendly ingredients into your meals.

How would you rate this dish?

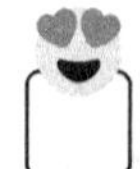 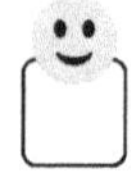  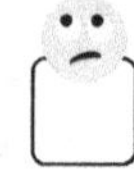 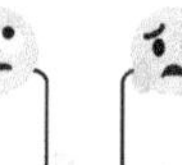 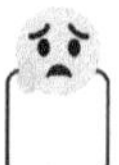

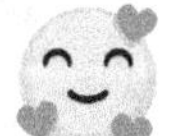 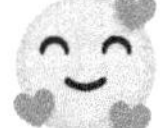 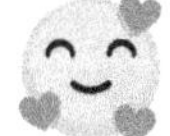 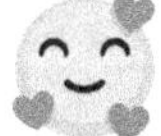 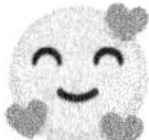 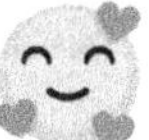 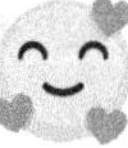 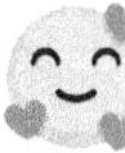 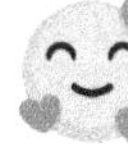 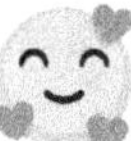

69. Sweet potato and black bean enchiladas

Let's do that and fill in the time here Prep Time :   Cook Time :   Servings :

Is this dish easy or difficult for you to make?

 ◯   ◯

Write 5 friends with whom you want to share this dish

....

....

....

....

....

INGREDIENTS

- 2 medium sweet potatoes, peeled and diced
- 1 (15 oz) can black beans, rinsed and drained
- 1 cup frozen corn kernels
- 1/2 cup diced onion
- 2 cloves garlic, minced
- 1 teaspoon ground cumin
- 1/2 teaspoon chili powder
- 1/4 teaspoon salt
- 8-10 corn tortillas
- 1 (15 oz) can enchilada sauce
- 1 cup shredded Monterey Jack or cheddar cheese

For Serving:
- Chopped fresh cilantro
- Diced avocado
- Lime wedges

1. Preheat oven to 375°F. Grease a 9x13-inch baking dish.

2. In a large skillet, sauté the diced sweet potatoes over medium heat for 5-7 minutes, until starting to soften.

3. Add the black beans, frozen corn, diced onion, and minced garlic to the skillet. Cook for 3-4 minutes, until the onion is translucent.

4. Stir in the cumin, chili powder, and salt. Remove from heat.

5. Spread 1/2 cup of the enchilada sauce in the bottom of the prepared baking dish.

6. Spoon about 1/4 cup of the sweet potato and black bean mixture onto each corn tortilla. Roll up the tortillas and place seam-side down in the baking dish.

7. Pour the remaining enchilada sauce over the top of the enchiladas and sprinkle with the shredded cheese.

8. Bake for 20-25 minutes, until the cheese is melted and bubbly.

9. Serve the enchiladas warm, topped with chopped cilantro, diced avocado, and lime wedges.

This sweet potato and black bean enchilada dish is an excellent choice for the MIND diet, as it features vegetables (sweet potatoes), legumes (black beans), and healthy fats (avocado). The combination of nutrients supports brain health and cognitive function, making it a great option for seniors over 60.

How would you rate this dish?

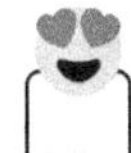 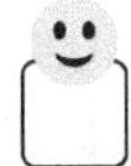 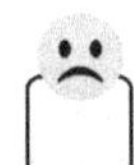 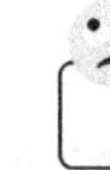 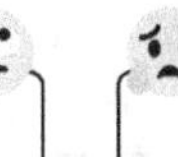 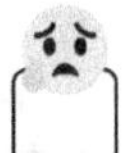

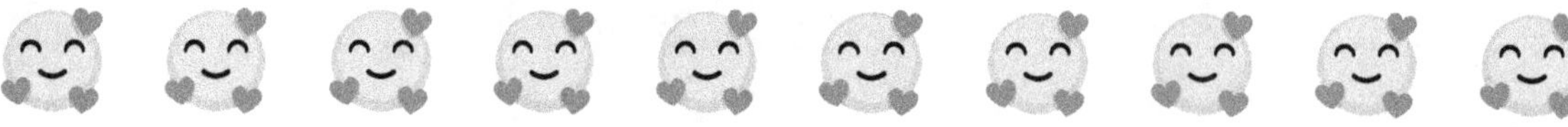

70. Spinach and ricotta stuffed shells

Let's do that and fill in the time here  Prep Time :   Cook Time :   Servings :

Is this dish easy or difficult for you to make?

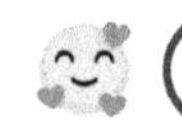 ◯   ◯

Write 5 friends with whom you want to share this dish

....

....

....

....

....

INGREDIENTS

- 12 jumbo pasta shells
- 1 (15 oz) container part-skim ricotta cheese
- 1 (10 oz) package frozen chopped spinach, thawed and squeezed dry
- 1 egg
- 1/4 cup grated Parmesan cheese
- 1 clove garlic, minced
- 1/4 teaspoon salt
- 1/4 teaspoon black pepper
- 1 (24 oz) jar marinara sauce
- 1 cup shredded mozzarella cheese

1. Preheat oven to 375°F. Grease a 9x13-inch baking dish.

2. Cook the pasta shells according to package instructions until al dente. Drain and set aside.

3. In a medium bowl, mix together the ricotta cheese, spinach, egg, Parmesan, garlic, salt, and pepper until well combined.

4. Stuff each cooked pasta shell with a heaping tablespoon of the ricotta-spinach mixture.

5. Spread 1/2 cup of the marinara sauce in the bottom of the prepared baking dish. Arrange the stuffed shells in a single layer.

6. Pour the remaining marinara sauce over the top of the shells, then sprinkle with the shredded mozzarella cheese.

7. Bake for 25-30 minutes, until the cheese is melted and bubbly.

8. Let the stuffed shells cool for 5 minutes before serving.

This dish is an excellent choice for the MIND diet, as it features whole grains (pasta shells), vegetables (spinach), and dairy (ricotta and mozzarella). The combination of nutrients supports brain health and cognitive function, making it a great option for seniors over 60.

Serve the spinach and ricotta stuffed shells with a side salad or steamed vegetables for a complete and balanced MIND diet-friendly meal.

How would you rate this dish?

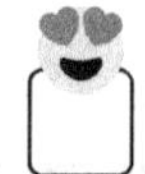 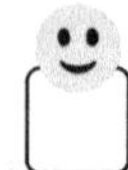 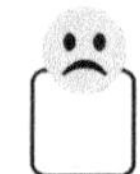 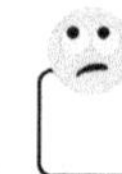 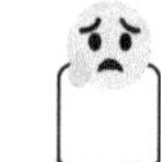

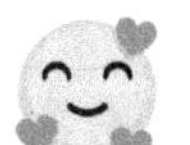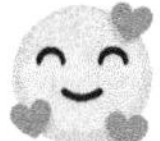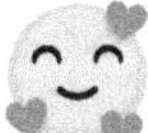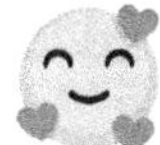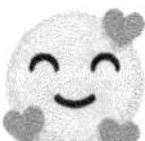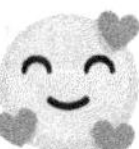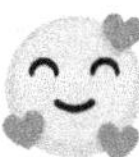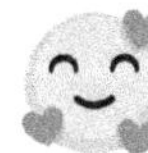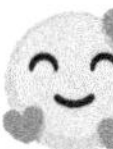

71. Baked tilapia with lemon and capers

Let's do that and fill in the time here 🕐 Prep Time :   🕐 Cook Time :   🍴 Servings :

Is this dish easy or difficult for you to make?

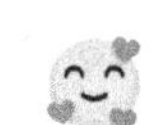 ◯   😊 ◯

Write 5 friends with whom you want to share this dish

....

....

....

....

....

INGREDIENTS

- 4 tilapia fillets (about 1 lb total)
- 2 tablespoons olive oil
- 2 tablespoons lemon juice
- 2 tablespoons capers, drained
- 2 cloves garlic, minced
- 1/4 teaspoon salt
- 1/4 teaspoon black pepper
- 2 tablespoons chopped fresh parsley

1. Preheat oven to 400°F. Grease a baking dish or line with parchment paper.

2. Place the tilapia fillets in the prepared baking dish.

3. In a small bowl, whisk together the olive oil, lemon juice, capers, garlic, salt, and black pepper.

4. Drizzle the lemon-caper mixture over the tilapia fillets, making sure to coat them evenly.

5. Bake for 15-18 minutes, until the fish flakes easily with a fork.

6. Remove the baked tilapia from the oven and sprinkle with the chopped fresh parsley.

7. Serve the tilapia warm, with the lemon-caper sauce spooned over the top.

This baked tilapia dish is an excellent choice for the MIND diet, as it features fatty fish (tilapia), healthy fats (olive oil), and herbs (parsley). The combination of nutrients supports brain health and cognitive function, making it a great option for seniors over 60.

Tilapia is a good source of omega-3 fatty acids, which are important for brain health. The lemon and capers add a bright, flavorful twist to the dish. Serve the baked tilapia with a side of roasted vegetables or a fresh salad for a complete MIND diet-friendly meal.

How would you rate this dish?

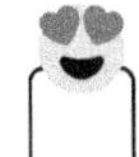 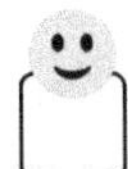 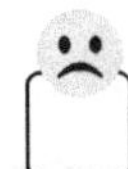 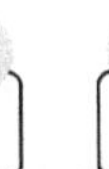 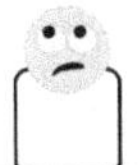 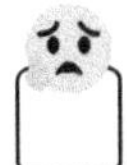

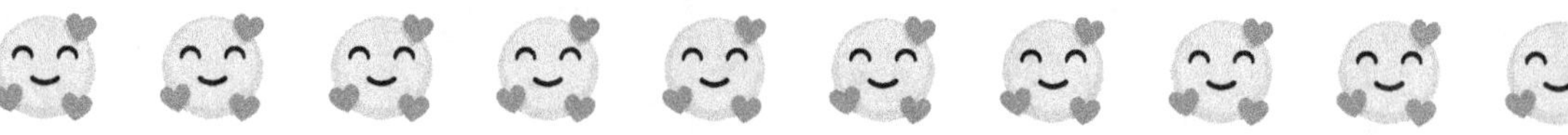

72. Grilled swordfish with a mango salsa

 Prep Time :   Cook Time :   Servings :

Is this dish easy or difficult for you to make?

 ⭕   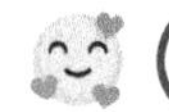 ⭕

Write 5 friends with whom you want to share this dish

....

....

....

....

INGREDIENTS

For the Mango Salsa:
- 1 ripe mango, diced
- 1/2 red onion, finely chopped
- 1 jalapeño, seeded and finely chopped
- 2 tablespoons chopped fresh cilantro
- 1 tablespoon lime juice
- 1/4 teaspoon salt

For the Swordfish:
- 4 (6 oz) swordfish steaks
- 1 tablespoon olive oil
- 1/2 teaspoon salt
- 1/4 teaspoon black pepper

1. Make the mango salsa: In a medium bowl, combine the diced mango, red onion, jalapeño, cilantro, lime juice, and salt. Stir to mix well and set aside.

2. Preheat grill or grill pan to medium-high heat.

3. Brush the swordfish steaks with the olive oil and season with salt and pepper.

4. Grill the swordfish for 4-5 minutes per side, or until it flakes easily with a fork.

5. Transfer the grilled swordfish to a serving platter and top with the prepared mango salsa.

6. Serve the swordfish and salsa immediately.

This grilled swordfish dish is an excellent choice for the MIND diet, as it features fatty fish (swordfish), fresh fruit (mango), and herbs (cilantro). The combination of nutrients supports brain health and cognitive function, making it a great option for seniors over 60.

Swordfish is a good source of omega-3 fatty acids, which are important for brain health. The mango salsa adds a sweet and tangy contrast to the savory fish, while the jalapeño provides a subtle heat.

Serve this grilled swordfish with a side of roasted vegetables or a fresh green salad for a complete MIND diet-friendly meal.

How would you rate this dish?

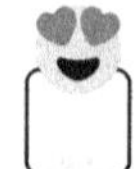 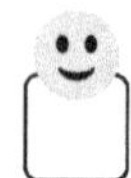 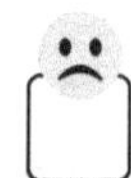 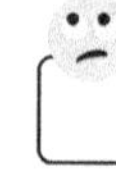 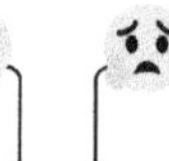

 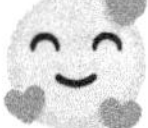 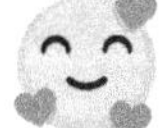 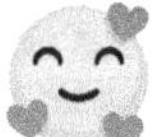 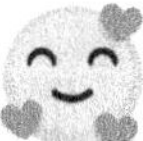 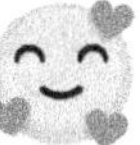 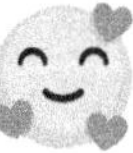 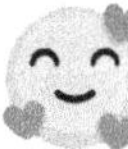 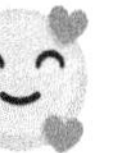 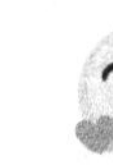

73. Shrimp and avocado salad

Let's do that and fill in the time here Prep Time :   Cook Time :   Servings :

Is this dish easy or difficult for you to make?

Write 5 friends with whom you want to share this dish
....
....
....
....
....

INGREDIENTS

- 1 lb cooked shrimp, peeled and deveined
- 2 avocados, diced
- 1 cup cherry tomatoes, halved
- 1/2 cup diced red onion
- 2 tablespoons chopped fresh cilantro
- 2 tablespoons olive oil
- 2 tablespoons lime juice
- 1/4 teaspoon salt
- 1/4 teaspoon black pepper

1. In a large bowl, gently combine the cooked shrimp, diced avocado, cherry tomatoes, red onion, and chopped cilantro.

2. In a small bowl, whisk together the olive oil, lime juice, salt, and black pepper.

3. Drizzle the dressing over the shrimp and avocado salad and toss gently to coat.

4. Serve the salad chilled or at room temperature.

This shrimp and avocado salad is an excellent choice for the MIND diet, as it features seafood (shrimp), healthy fats (avocado, olive oil), and vegetables (tomatoes, onion, cilantro). The combination of nutrients supports brain health and cognitive function, making it a great option for seniors over 60.

Shrimp is a good source of lean protein, while avocado provides heart-healthy monounsaturated fats. The fresh lime juice and cilantro add a bright, refreshing flavor to the salad.

Serve this salad on its own or over a bed of mixed greens for a light and nutritious MIND diet-friendly meal.

How would you rate this dish?

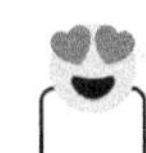 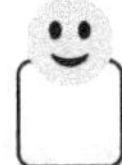 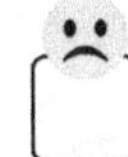 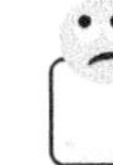 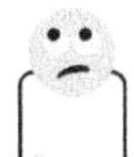 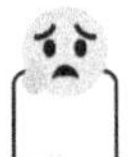

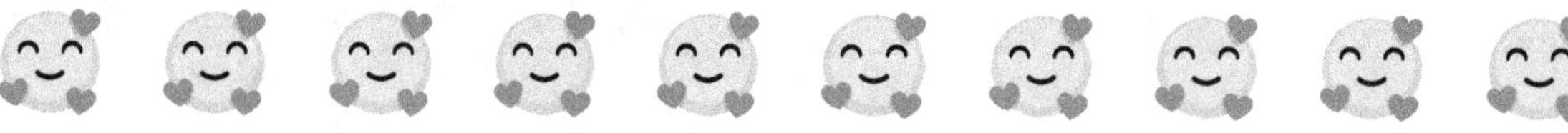

74. Baked haddock with a breadcrumb crust

 Prep Time :   Cook Time :   Servings :

Is this dish easy or difficult for you to make?

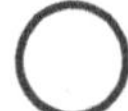 ◯   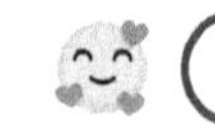 ◯

Write 5 friends with whom you want to share this dish

....

....

....

....

....

INGREDIENTS

- 4 (6 oz) haddock fillets
- 1/2 cup panko breadcrumbs
- 2 tablespoons grated Parmesan cheese
- 2 tablespoons chopped fresh parsley
- 1 tablespoon olive oil
- 1/4 teaspoon salt
- 1/4 teaspoon black pepper

1. Preheat oven to 400°F. Grease a baking dish or line with parchment paper.

2. In a shallow bowl, mix together the panko breadcrumbs, Parmesan cheese, parsley, olive oil, salt, and pepper.

3. Place the haddock fillets in the prepared baking dish. Evenly top each fillet with the breadcrumb mixture, pressing it down gently to adhere.

4. Bake for 15-18 minutes, until the fish is opaque and flakes easily with a fork, and the breadcrumb topping is golden brown.

5. Serve the baked haddock immediately, garnished with additional chopped parsley if desired.

This baked haddock dish is an excellent choice for the MIND diet, as it features fatty fish (haddock), whole grains (panko breadcrumbs), and herbs (parsley). The combination of nutrients supports brain health and cognitive function, making it a great option for seniors over 60.

Haddock is a good source of omega-3 fatty acids, which are important for brain health. The breadcrumb topping adds a nice crunch and texture to the dish, while the Parmesan cheese and parsley provide additional flavor.

Serve the baked haddock with a side of roasted vegetables or a fresh salad for a complete MIND diet-friendly meal.

How would you rate this dish?

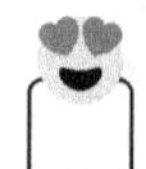 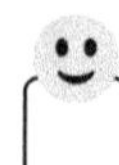 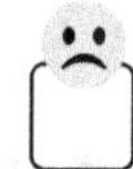 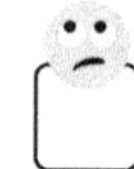 

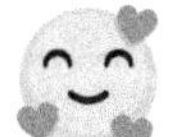 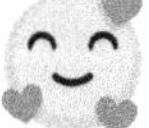 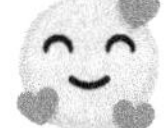 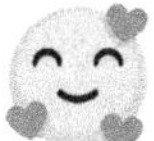 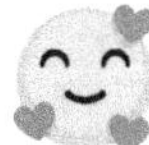 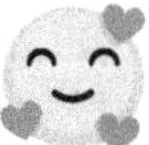 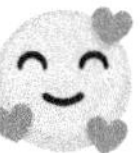 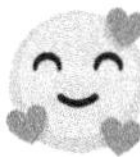 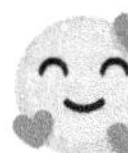 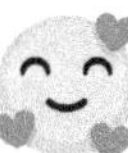

75. Sardine and arugula salad

Prep Time :   Cook Time :   Servings :

Is this dish easy or difficult for you to make?

 ◯    ◯

Write 5 friends with whom you want to share this dish

....

....

....

....

....

INGREDIENTS

- 4 cups baby arugula
- 1 (4 oz) can sardines in olive oil, drained and flaked
- 1 avocado, diced
- 1/4 cup sliced red onion
- 2 tablespoons toasted pine nuts
- 2 tablespoons balsamic vinegar
- 1 tablespoon extra-virgin olive oil
- 1/4 teaspoon salt
- 1/4 teaspoon black pepper

1. In a large salad bowl, combine the baby arugula, flaked sardines, diced avocado, and sliced red onion.

2. In a small bowl, whisk together the balsamic vinegar, olive oil, salt, and black pepper.

3. Drizzle the dressing over the salad and toss gently to coat.

4. Sprinkle the toasted pine nuts over the top of the salad.

5. Serve immediately.

This sardine and arugula salad is a nutritious and flavorful option. Sardines are an excellent source of omega-3 fatty acids, which are important for brain health. The peppery arugula, creamy avocado, and crunchy pine nuts provide a variety of textures and flavors.

The balsamic vinaigrette dressing ties all the ingredients together nicely. This salad makes a great light meal or side dish.

For a MIND diet-friendly version, be sure to use extra-virgin olive oil in the dressing, as it is a healthy fat that supports brain function. Enjoy this delicious and nutrient-dense salad!

How would you rate this dish?

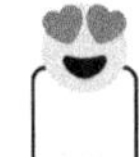 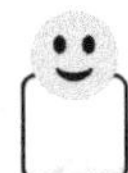 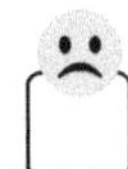 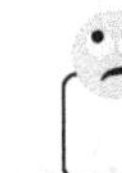 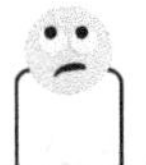 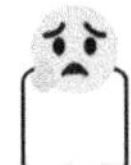

76. Mackerel with a tomato and onion relish

 Prep Time :   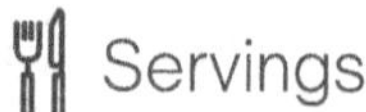 Cook Time :   Servings :

Is this dish easy or difficult for you to make?

○   ○

Write 5 friends with whom you want to share this dish ....

INGREDIENTS

For the Relish:
- 2 cups diced tomatoes
- 1/2 cup diced red onion
- 2 tablespoons chopped fresh parsley
- 1 tablespoon red wine vinegar
- 1 tablespoon olive oil
- 1/4 teaspoon salt
- 1/4 teaspoon black pepper

For the Mackerel:
- 4 (6 oz) mackerel fillets
- 1 tablespoon olive oil
- 1/2 teaspoon salt
- 1/4 teaspoon black pepper

1. Make the relish: In a medium bowl, combine the diced tomatoes, red onion, parsley, red wine vinegar, olive oil, salt, and pepper. Stir to mix well and set aside.

2. Preheat grill or grill pan to medium-high heat.

3. Brush the mackerel fillets with the olive oil and season with salt and pepper.

4. Grill the mackerel for 3-4 minutes per side, until cooked through and flaky.

5. Transfer the grilled mackerel to a serving platter and top with the tomato and onion relish.

6. Serve the mackerel immediately, with the relish spooned over the top.

Mackerel is an oily, fatty fish that is rich in omega-3 fatty acids, which are beneficial for brain health. The tomato and onion relish provides a fresh, tangy contrast to the rich mackerel.

This dish is a great option for the MIND diet, as it features fatty fish, vegetables, and healthy fats. Serve it with a side of roasted vegetables or a simple salad for a complete and nutritious meal.

How would you rate this dish?

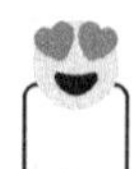 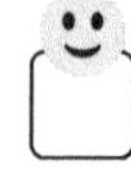 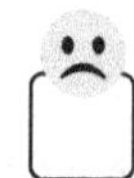 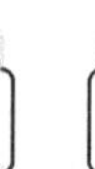 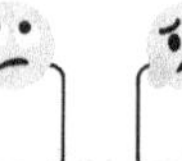 

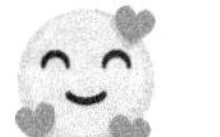 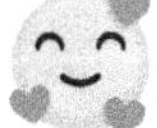 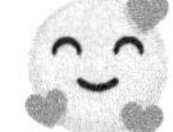 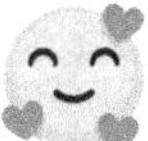 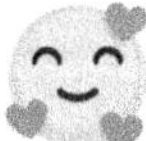 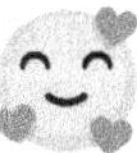 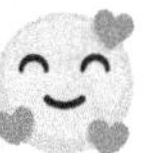 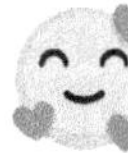  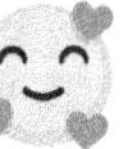 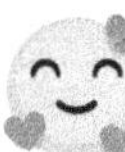

77. Tuna steak with a wasabi glaze

Let's do that and fill in the time here 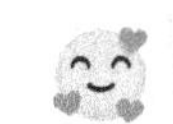 Prep Time :   Cook Time :   Servings :

Is this dish easy or difficult for you to make?

😰 ◯   😊 ◯

Write 5 friends with whom you want to share this dish

....
....
....
....
....

INGREDIENTS

- 4 (6 oz) tuna steaks
- 2 tablespoons soy sauce
- 1 tablespoon rice vinegar
- 1 tablespoon honey
- 1 tablespoon wasabi paste
- 1 teaspoon sesame oil
- 1/4 teaspoon salt
- 1/4 teaspoon black pepper
- 2 tablespoons sesame seeds
- 2 tablespoons chopped fresh cilantro (optional)

1. In a small bowl, whisk together the soy sauce, rice vinegar, honey, wasabi paste, and sesame oil. Set aside.

2. Season the tuna steaks with salt and pepper on both sides.

3. Heat a grill or grill pan over medium-high heat. Grill the tuna steaks for 2-3 minutes per side, or until cooked to your desired doneness.

4. Transfer the grilled tuna steaks to a plate and brush them generously with the wasabi glaze.

5. Sprinkle the sesame seeds over the top of the tuna steaks.

6. Garnish with chopped fresh cilantro, if desired.

7. Serve the tuna steaks immediately.

This tuna dish is an excellent choice for the MIND diet, as it features fatty fish (tuna), healthy fats (sesame oil), and herbs (cilantro). The combination of nutrients supports brain health and cognitive function, making it a great option for seniors over 60.

Tuna is a rich source of omega-3 fatty acids, which are important for brain health. The wasabi glaze adds a flavorful kick, while the sesame seeds provide a nice crunch.

Serve the tuna steaks with a side of steamed vegetables or a fresh salad for a complete MIND diet-friendly meal.

How would you rate this dish?

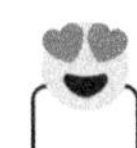 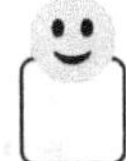  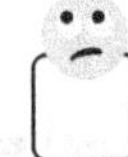 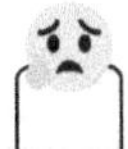

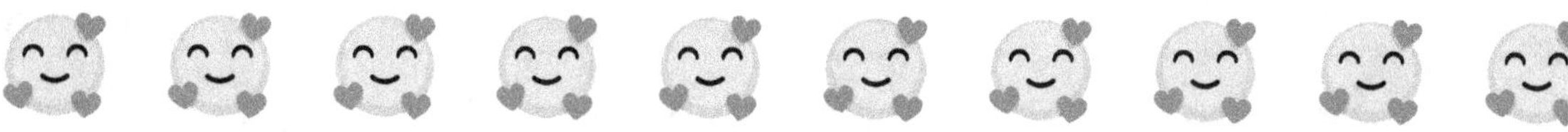

78. Salmon cakes with a dill yogurt sauce

 Prep Time :   Cook Time :   Servings :

Is this dish easy or difficult for you to make?

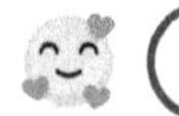 ◯   ◯

Write 5 friends with whom you want to share this dish

....

....

....

....

....

INGREDIENTS

For the Salmon Cakes:
- 1 (15 oz) can wild-caught salmon, drained and flaked
- 1 egg, lightly beaten
- 1/2 cup whole wheat breadcrumbs
- 2 tablespoons chopped fresh parsley
- 1 tablespoon Dijon mustard
- 1/4 teaspoon salt
- 1/4 teaspoon black pepper
- 1 tablespoon olive oil

For the Dill Yogurt Sauce:
- 1 cup plain Greek yogurt
- 2 tablespoons chopped fresh dill
- 1 tablespoon lemon juice
- 1/4 teaspoon salt

1. In a medium bowl, gently mix together the flaked salmon, egg, breadcrumbs, parsley, Dijon mustard, salt, and pepper until well combined.

2. Form the mixture into 8 small patties, about 1/2 inch thick.

3. In a large skillet, heat the olive oil over medium heat. Cook the salmon cakes for 3-4 minutes per side, until golden brown.

4. In a small bowl, mix together the Greek yogurt, chopped dill, lemon juice, and salt for the dill yogurt sauce.

5. Serve the warm salmon cakes with the dill yogurt sauce on the side.

This salmon cake dish is an excellent choice for the MIND diet, as it features fatty fish (salmon), dairy (yogurt), and herbs (parsley, dill). The combination of nutrients supports brain health and cognitive function, making it a great option for seniors over 60.

Salmon is a rich source of omega-3 fatty acids, which are important for brain health. The whole wheat breadcrumbs and Greek yogurt also provide additional nutrients that are beneficial for the MIND diet.

Serve the salmon cakes with a side of roasted vegetables or a fresh salad for a complete and balanced meal.

How would you rate this dish?

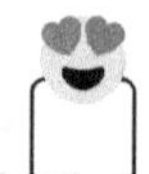 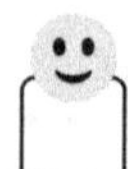 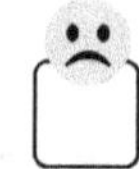 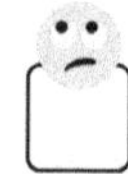 

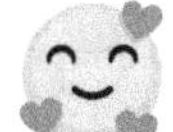 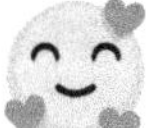 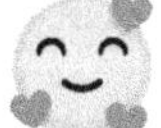 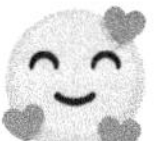 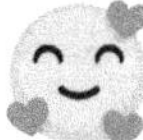 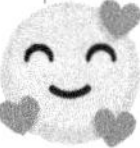 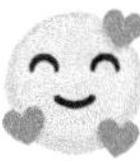 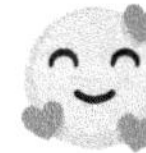  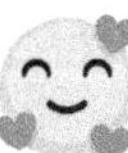

79. Crab-stuffed mushrooms

Let's do that and fill in the time here 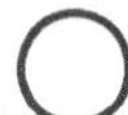 Prep Time :   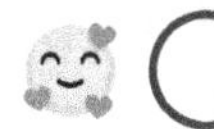 Cook Time :   Servings :

Is this dish easy or difficult for you to make?

Write 5 friends with whom you want to share this dish

....
....
....
....
....

INGREDIENTS

- 12 large button or cremini mushrooms, stems removed and finely chopped
- 1 tablespoon olive oil
- 2 cloves garlic, minced
- 1/4 cup finely chopped onion
- 1 (6 oz) can lump crabmeat, drained and flaked
- 2 tablespoons grated Parmesan cheese
- 2 tablespoons panko breadcrumbs
- 1 tablespoon chopped fresh parsley
- 1/4 teaspoon salt
- 1/4 teaspoon black pepper

1. Preheat oven to 375°F. Grease a baking sheet or line with parchment paper.

2. In a skillet, heat the olive oil over medium heat. Add the chopped mushroom stems, garlic, and onion. Sauté for 3-4 minutes, until the vegetables are softened.

3. Remove the skillet from heat and stir in the crabmeat, Parmesan cheese, panko breadcrumbs, parsley, salt, and pepper until well combined.

4. Spoon the crab mixture evenly into the mushroom caps, packing it in gently.

5. Arrange the stuffed mushrooms on the prepared baking sheet.

6. Bake for 12-15 minutes, until the mushrooms are tender and the filling is hot and bubbly.

7. Serve the crab-stuffed mushrooms warm.

This appetizer is an excellent choice for the MIND diet, as it features seafood (crabmeat), dairy (Parmesan), and herbs (parsley). The combination of nutrients supports brain health and cognitive function, making it a great option for seniors over 60.

Crabmeat is a good source of lean protein, while the Parmesan cheese and panko breadcrumbs add a nice texture and flavor to the filling. The mushrooms themselves also provide additional nutrients.

These crab-stuffed mushrooms make a delicious and MIND diet-friendly hors d'oeuvre or side dish.

How would you rate this dish?

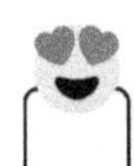 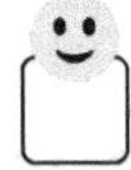  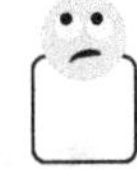 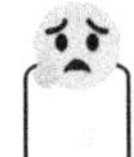

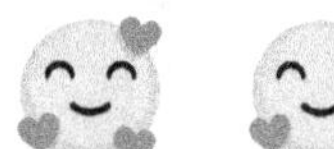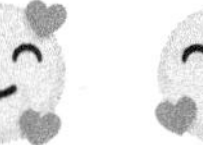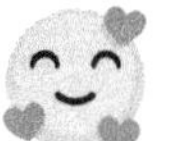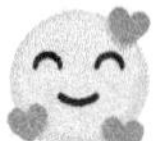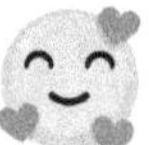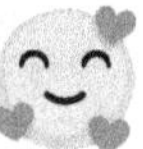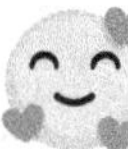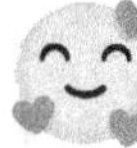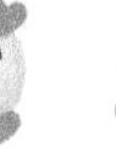

80. Seafood paella

Let's do that and fill in the time here ✅ Prep Time : 🕐 Cook Time : 🍴 Servings :

Is this dish easy or difficult for you to make?

😭 ◯　　　 ◯

Write 5 friends with whom you want to share this dish

....
....
....
....
....

INGREDIENTS

- 2 tablespoons olive oil
- 1 onion, diced
- 3 cloves garlic, minced
- 1 cup short-grain Spanish rice (such as Bomba or Calasparra)
- 1 teaspoon smoked paprika
- 1/2 teaspoon saffron threads
- 1 cup dry white wine
- 2 cups seafood or chicken broth
- 1 lb large shrimp, peeled and deveined
- 1 lb mussels, scrubbed and debearded
- 1 lb calamari, bodies sliced into rings and tentacles left whole
- 1 cup frozen peas
- 1 lemon, cut into wedges for serving
- Salt and pepper to taste

1. In a large paella pan or deep skillet, heat the olive oil over medium-high heat. Add the onion and sauté for 3-4 minutes until translucent.

2. Stir in the garlic and cook for 1 minute until fragrant.

3. Add the rice, smoked paprika, and saffron. Stir to coat the rice with the spices and oil.

4. Pour in the white wine and let it simmer for 2-3 minutes until mostly absorbed.

5. Add the seafood broth and bring the mixture to a boil. Reduce heat to medium-low, cover, and simmer for 15-18 minutes, until the rice is tender and has absorbed most of the liquid.

6. Uncover and arrange the shrimp, mussels, and calamari over the top of the rice. Cover and cook for 5-7 minutes, until the seafood is cooked through.

7. Stir in the frozen peas and season with salt and pepper to taste.

8. Serve the seafood paella immediately, garnished with lemon wedges.

This classic Spanish dish is a delicious way to enjoy a variety of fresh seafood. The saffron and smoked paprika give the paella its signature flavor and vibrant color. Enjoy this hearty and flavorful meal!

How would you rate this dish?

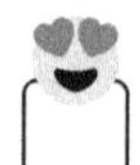 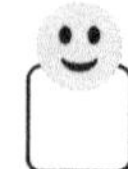 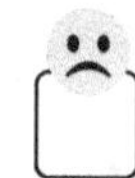 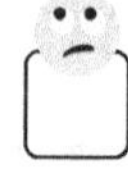 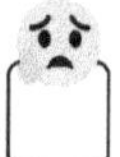

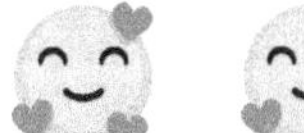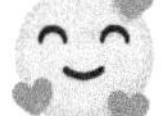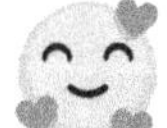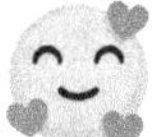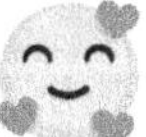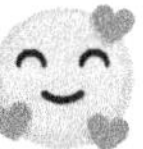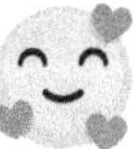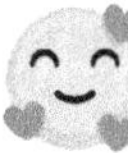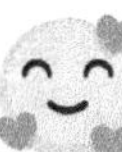

81. Roast chicken with rosemary and garlic

 Prep Time :   Cook Time :   Servings :

Is this dish easy or difficult for you to make?

Write 5 friends with whom you want to share this dish

....
....
....
....
....

INGREDIENTS

- 1 (4-5 lb) whole chicken
- 3 tablespoons olive oil
- 4 cloves garlic, minced
- 2 tablespoons chopped fresh rosemary
- 1 teaspoon salt
- 1/2 teaspoon black pepper
- 1 lemon, cut into wedges

1. Preheat oven to 400°F. Grease a large roasting pan or baking dish.

2. Pat the chicken dry with paper towels. Rub the skin all over with 2 tablespoons of the olive oil.

3. In a small bowl, mix together the minced garlic, chopped rosemary, salt, and pepper. Rub this seasoning mixture all over the chicken, including under the skin.

4. Place the chicken in the prepared roasting pan. Tuck the lemon wedges around the chicken.

5. Roast the chicken for 1 to 1 1/2 hours, until the juices run clear when the thigh is pierced with a fork and the internal temperature reaches 165°F.

6. Baste the chicken with the remaining 1 tablespoon of olive oil halfway through the cooking time.

7. Let the chicken rest for 10 minutes before carving and serving.

This roast chicken dish is an excellent choice for the MIND diet, as it features lean protein (chicken), herbs (rosemary), and healthy fats (olive oil). The combination of nutrients supports brain health and cognitive function, making it a great option for seniors over 60.

Chicken is a good source of protein, while the rosemary and garlic add flavor and antioxidants. The lemon wedges provide a bright, refreshing contrast.

Serve the roast chicken with a side of roasted vegetables or a fresh salad for a complete MIND diet-friendly meal.

How would you rate this dish?

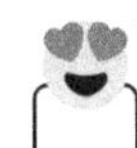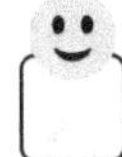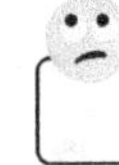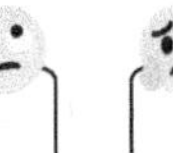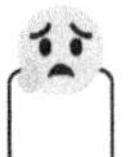

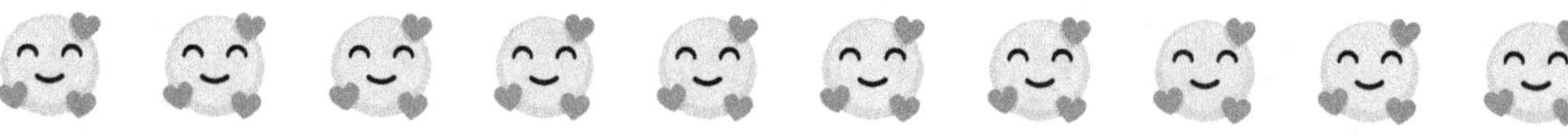

82. Chicken stir-fry with broccoli and cashews

 Prep Time :　　Cook Time :　　Servings :

Is this dish easy or difficult for you to make?

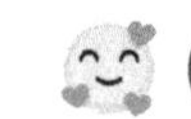 ◯　　　◯

Write 5 friends with whom you want to share this dish
....
....
....
....
....

INGREDIENTS

- 1 lb boneless, skinless chicken breasts, cut into 1-inch pieces
- 2 tablespoons low-sodium soy sauce
- 1 tablespoon rice vinegar
- 1 teaspoon sesame oil
- 2 tablespoons olive oil
- 3 cups broccoli florets
- 1 red bell pepper, sliced
- 3 cloves garlic, minced
- 1 tablespoon grated fresh ginger
- 1/2 cup unsalted roasted cashews
- 2 cups cooked brown rice, for serving

1. In a medium bowl, combine the chicken, soy sauce, rice vinegar, and sesame oil. Toss to coat the chicken and let marinate for 15 minutes.

2. Heat the olive oil in a large skillet or wok over high heat. Add the marinated chicken and stir-fry for 3-4 minutes, until lightly browned.

3. Add the broccoli florets and red bell pepper to the skillet. Stir-fry for 3-4 minutes, until the vegetables are crisp-tender.

4. Stir in the minced garlic and grated ginger. Cook for 1 minute, until fragrant.

5. Remove the skillet from heat and stir in the roasted cashews.

6. Serve the chicken stir-fry immediately over the cooked brown rice.

This chicken stir-fry is an excellent choice for the MIND diet, as it features lean protein (chicken), vegetables (broccoli, bell pepper), healthy fats (olive oil, cashews), and whole grains (brown rice). The combination of nutrients supports brain health and cognitive function, making it a great option for seniors over 60.

The soy sauce, rice vinegar, and sesame oil provide a flavorful Asian-inspired sauce, while the cashews add a satisfying crunch.

Serve this stir-fry with a side of steamed greens or a fresh salad for a complete MIND diet-friendly meal.

How would you rate this dish?

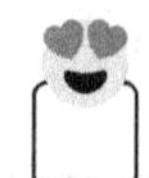 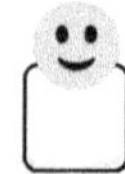 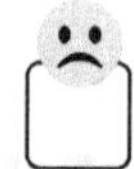 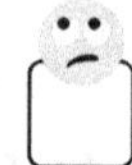 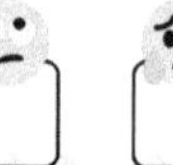 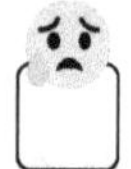

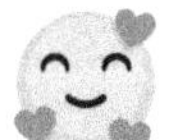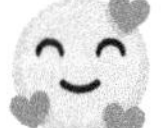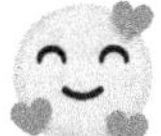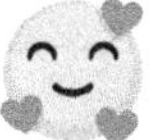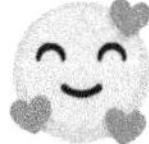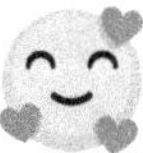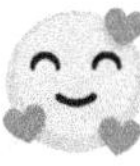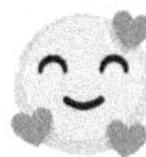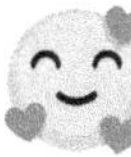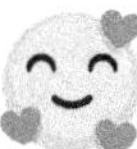

83. Turkey meatballs with a marinara sauce

Let's do that and fill in the time here 🕤 Prep Time :   🕐 Cook Time :   🍴 Servings :

Is this dish easy or difficult for you to make?

 ◯    ◯

Write 5 friends with whom you want to share this dish ....

INGREDIENTS

For the Meatballs:
- 1 lb ground turkey
- 1/2 cup whole wheat breadcrumbs
- 1/4 cup grated Parmesan cheese
- 1 egg, lightly beaten
- 2 cloves garlic, minced
- 2 tablespoons chopped fresh parsley
- 1/2 teaspoon salt
- 1/4 teaspoon black pepper

For the Marinara Sauce:
- 1 tablespoon olive oil
- 1 onion, diced
- 3 cloves garlic, minced
- 1 (28 oz) can crushed tomatoes
- 2 tablespoons tomato paste
- 1 teaspoon dried oregano
- 1/4 teaspoon red pepper flakes (optional)
- Salt and pepper to taste

1. Preheat oven to 400°F. Line a baking sheet with parchment paper.

2. In a large bowl, combine all the meatball ingredients and mix well until just combined. Roll the mixture into 1-inch meatballs and place them on the prepared baking sheet.

3. Bake the meatballs for 18-20 minutes, until cooked through.

4. While the meatballs are baking, make the marinara sauce. In a saucepan, heat the olive oil over medium heat. Add the onion and sauté for 3-4 minutes until translucent.

5. Stir in the garlic and cook for 1 minute until fragrant.

6. Add the crushed tomatoes, tomato paste, oregano, and red pepper flakes (if using). Season with salt and pepper to taste.

7. Simmer the marinara sauce for 10-15 minutes, stirring occasionally, until thickened.

8. Add the cooked meatballs to the marinara sauce and gently toss to coat.

9. Serve the turkey meatballs and sauce over a bed of whole wheat pasta or zucchini noodles.

This turkey meatball dish is an excellent choice for the MIND diet, as it features lean protein (turkey), whole grains (whole wheat breadcrumbs and pasta), vegetables (tomatoes, onion, garlic), and herbs (parsley, oregano). The combination of nutrients supports brain health and cognitive function, making it a great option for seniors over 60.

How would you rate this dish?

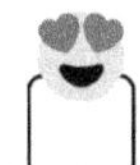 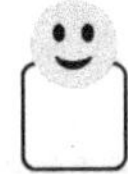 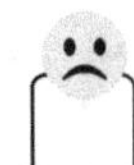  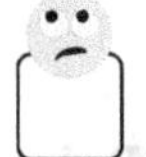 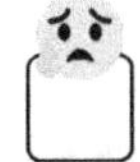

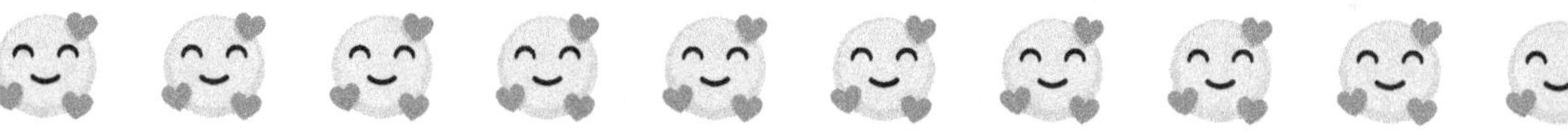

84. Chicken fajitas with bell peppers

Let's do that and fill in the time here  Prep Time :   Cook Time :   Servings :

Is this dish easy or difficult for you to make?

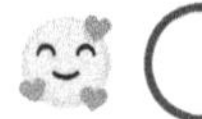 ◯   ◯

Write 5 friends with whom you want to share this dish

....

....

....

....

INGREDIENTS

- 1 lb boneless, skinless chicken breasts, sliced into thin strips
- 2 tablespoons olive oil
- 1 tablespoon chili powder
- 1 teaspoon ground cumin
- 1/2 teaspoon garlic powder
- 1/4 teaspoon salt
- 1/4 teaspoon black pepper
- 2 bell peppers (any color), sliced into thin strips
- 1 onion, sliced
- 8-10 whole wheat tortillas
- Toppings: diced avocado, salsa, plain Greek yogurt, chopped cilantro

1. In a large bowl, toss the chicken strips with 1 tablespoon of the olive oil, chili powder, cumin, garlic powder, salt, and pepper until well coated.

2. Heat the remaining 1 tablespoon of olive oil in a large skillet or wok over medium-high heat. Add the seasoned chicken and cook for 5-7 minutes, stirring occasionally, until the chicken is cooked through.

3. Add the sliced bell peppers and onion to the skillet. Sauté for 5-7 minutes, until the vegetables are tender-crisp.

4. Warm the whole wheat tortillas according to package instructions.

5. To serve, place some of the chicken and vegetable mixture into each tortilla. Top with diced avocado, salsa, Greek yogurt, and chopped cilantro.

This chicken fajita dish is an excellent choice for the MIND diet, as it features lean protein (chicken), vegetables (bell peppers, onion), healthy fats (avocado, olive oil), and whole grains (whole wheat tortillas). The combination of nutrients supports brain health and cognitive function, making it a great option for seniors over 60.

The chili powder, cumin, and garlic add flavor to the chicken, while the toppings provide additional nutrients and textures. Serve this dish with a side of roasted sweet potatoes or a fresh salad for a complete MIND diet-friendly meal.

How would you rate this dish?

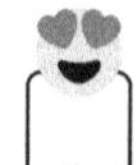 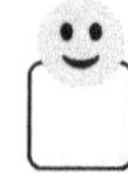   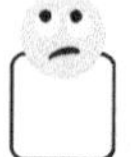 

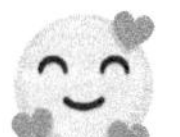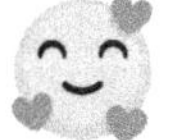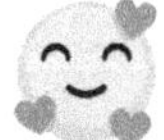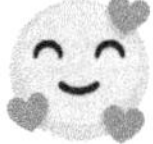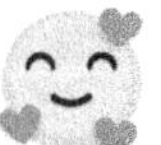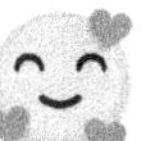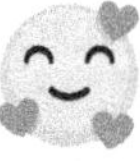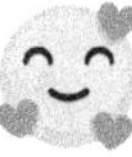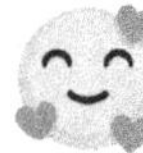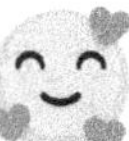

85. Grilled turkey burgers with avocado

Let's do that and fill in the time here Prep Time :   Cook Time :   Servings :

Is this dish easy or difficult for you to make?

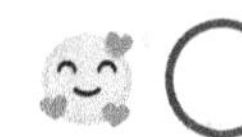

Write 5 friends with whom you want to share this dish

....

....

....

....

INGREDIENTS

- 1 lb ground turkey
- 1 tsp garlic powder
- 1 tsp onion powder
- 1 tsp dried oregano
- 1/2 tsp salt
- 1/4 tsp black pepper
- 1 avocado, sliced
- 4 whole wheat burger buns

1. In a large bowl, combine the ground turkey, garlic powder, onion powder, oregano, salt, and pepper. Mix well until the seasonings are evenly distributed.

2. Divide the turkey mixture into 4 equal portions and shape into patties, about 4-5 inches wide and 1/2 inch thick.

3. Preheat grill or grill pan to medium-high heat. Grill the turkey burgers for 4-5 minutes per side, or until cooked through and no longer pink in the center.

4. Place the grilled turkey burgers on the buns and top each one with sliced avocado.

5. Serve immediately and enjoy!

You can customize these turkey burgers by adding other toppings like tomato, onion, lettuce, or your favorite condiments. The avocado adds a creamy, healthy element to these lean turkey burgers.

How would you rate this dish?

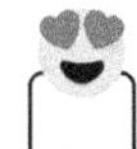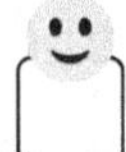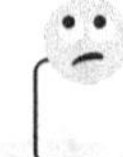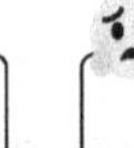

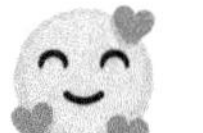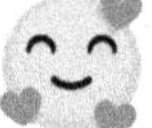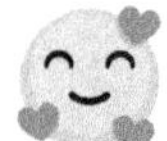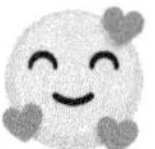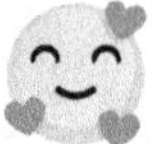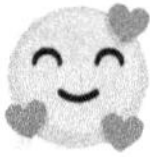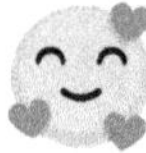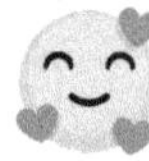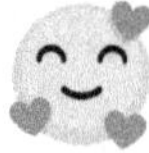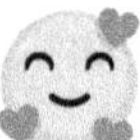

86. Lemon herb chicken breasts

Let's do that and fill in the time here **Prep Time :**   **Cook Time :**   **Servings :**

Is this dish easy or difficult for you to make?

 ○   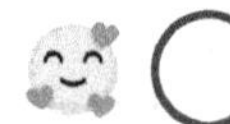 ○

Write 5 ....
friends
with ....
whom
you ....
want to
share ....
this
dish ....

INGREDIENTS

- 4 boneless, skinless chicken breasts
- 2 tbsp olive oil
- 2 tbsp fresh lemon juice
- 1 tsp dried oregano
- 1 tsp dried basil
- 1 tsp garlic powder
- 1/2 tsp salt
- 1/4 tsp black pepper

How would you rate this dish?

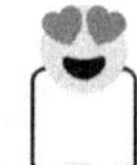 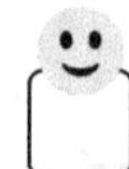 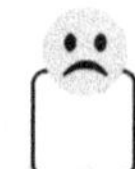 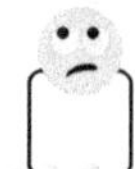 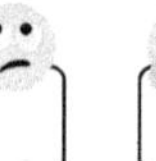 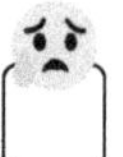

1. In a shallow baking dish or resealable plastic bag, combine the olive oil, lemon juice, oregano, basil, garlic powder, salt, and pepper. Add the chicken breasts and turn to coat evenly.

2. Cover the dish or seal the bag and marinate the chicken in the refrigerator for 30 minutes to 1 hour.

3. Preheat the oven to 400°F (200°C).

4. Remove the chicken from the marinade and place in a baking dish or on a rimmed baking sheet.

5. Bake the chicken for 20-25 minutes, or until it is cooked through and reaches an internal temperature of 165°F (75°C).

6. Serve the lemon herb chicken breasts immediately.

This recipe is MIND diet-friendly for seniors over 60 because it:

- Uses lean protein from chicken, which is recommended in the MIND diet.
- Includes healthy fats from olive oil.
- Features herbs and lemon, which are part of the MIND diet's emphasis on plant-based foods.
- Avoids processed ingredients and focuses on whole, unprocessed foods.

The MIND diet has been shown to help reduce the risk of cognitive decline and Alzheimer's disease in older adults. Enjoy this flavorful and nutritious lemon herb chicken as part of a MIND diet-friendly meal plan.

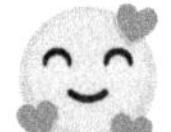 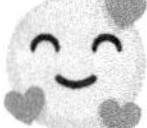 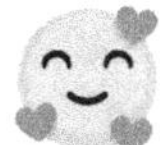 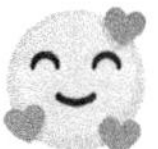 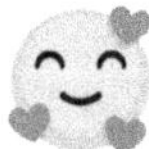 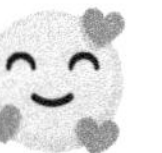 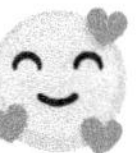 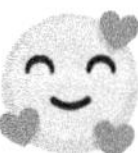 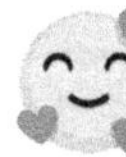 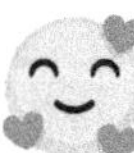

87. Chicken and chickpea stew

Let's do that and fill in the time here ◷ Prep Time :   ◷ Cook Time :   Servings :

Is this dish easy or difficult for you to make?

 ◯   ◯

Write 5 friends with whom you want to share this dish ....

INGREDIENTS

- 1 lb boneless, skinless chicken thighs, cut into 1-inch pieces
- 1 tbsp olive oil
- 1 onion, diced
- 3 cloves garlic, minced
- 2 carrots, peeled and sliced
- 2 celery stalks, sliced
- 1 tsp dried thyme
- 1 tsp dried rosemary
- 1 tsp paprika
- 1/2 tsp salt
- 1/4 tsp black pepper
- 1 (15 oz) can chickpeas, drained and rinsed
- 4 cups low-sodium chicken broth
- 2 cups baby spinach

How would you rate this dish?

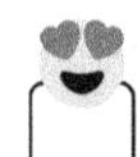 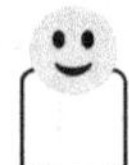  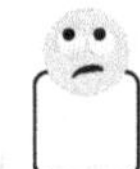 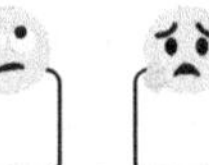 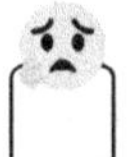

1. In a large pot or Dutch oven, heat the olive oil over medium-high heat. Add the chicken and cook for 3-4 minutes, until lightly browned.

2. Add the onion, garlic, carrots, and celery to the pot. Cook for 5-7 minutes, stirring occasionally, until the vegetables are softened.

3. Stir in the thyme, rosemary, paprika, salt, and pepper. Cook for 1 minute to toast the spices.

4. Add the chickpeas and chicken broth to the pot. Bring the mixture to a boil, then reduce the heat and simmer for 20-25 minutes, until the chicken is cooked through and the vegetables are tender.

5. Stir in the baby spinach and cook for 2-3 minutes, until the spinach is wilted.

6. Serve the chicken and chickpea stew hot.

This recipe supports the MIND diet for seniors over 60 because it:

- Uses lean protein from chicken, which is recommended in the MIND diet.
- Includes chickpeas, which are a legume and part of the MIND diet's emphasis on plant-based foods.
- Features vegetables like carrots, celery, and spinach, which are also key components of the MIND diet.
- Avoids processed ingredients and focuses on whole, unprocessed foods.

The MIND diet has been shown to help reduce the risk of cognitive decline and Alzheimer's disease in older adults. Enjoy this nourishing and flavorful chicken and chickpea stew as part of a MIND diet-friendly meal plan.

88. BBQ chicken with a side of coleslaw

 Prep Time :　　　Cook Time :　　　Servings :

Is this dish easy or difficult for you to make?

 ◯　　　😊 ◯

Write 5 ....
friends
with ....
whom
you ....
want to
share ....
this
dish ....

INGREDIENTS

For the BBQ Chicken:
- 4 boneless, skinless chicken breasts
- 1/2 cup barbecue sauce (look for one low in added sugars)
- 1 tsp smoked paprika
- 1/2 tsp garlic powder
- 1/4 tsp salt
- 1/4 tsp black pepper

For the Coleslaw:
- 3 cups shredded green cabbage
- 1 cup shredded red cabbage
- 1 carrot, grated
- 2 tbsp plain Greek yogurt
- 1 tbsp apple cider vinegar
- 1 tsp Dijon mustard
- 1 tsp honey
- 1/4 tsp salt
- 1/4 tsp black pepper

How would you rate this dish?

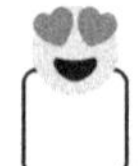 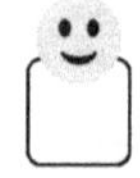   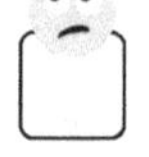 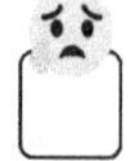

1. Preheat the oven to 400°F (200°C).

2. In a small bowl, mix together the barbecue sauce, smoked paprika, garlic powder, salt, and pepper. Place the chicken breasts in a baking dish and brush them evenly with the barbecue sauce mixture.

3. Bake the chicken for 25-30 minutes, or until it reaches an internal temperature of 165°F (75°C).

4. While the chicken is baking, prepare the coleslaw. In a large bowl, combine the shredded green cabbage, red cabbage, and grated carrot.

5. In a small bowl, whisk together the Greek yogurt, apple cider vinegar, Dijon mustard, honey, salt, and pepper.

6. Pour the dressing over the cabbage mixture and toss to coat evenly.

7. Serve the BBQ chicken with the coleslaw on the side.

This recipe supports the MIND diet for seniors over 60 because it:

- Uses lean protein from chicken, which is recommended in the MIND diet.
- Features a vegetable-based coleslaw with cabbage and carrots, which are part of the MIND diet's emphasis on plant-based foods.
- Includes healthy fats from the Greek yogurt in the coleslaw dressing.
- Avoids processed ingredients and focuses on whole, unprocessed foods.

The MIND diet has been shown to help reduce the risk of cognitive decline and Alzheimer's disease in older adults. Enjoy this delicious and nutritious BBQ chicken with coleslaw as part of a MIND diet-friendly meal plan.

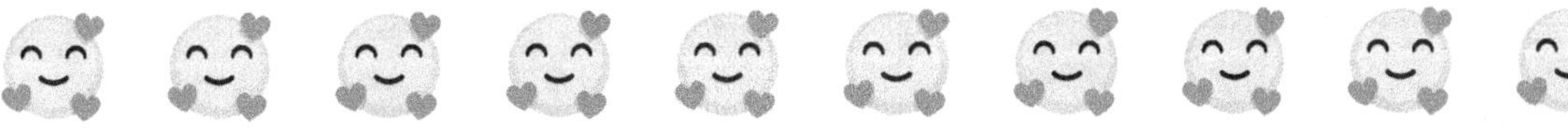

89. Stuffed chicken breast with spinach and feta

Let's do that and fill in the time here  Prep Time :   Cook Time :   Servings :

Is this dish easy or difficult for you to make?

Write 5 friends with whom you want to share this dish

....

....

....

....

....

INGREDIENTS

- 4 boneless, skinless chicken breasts
- 2 cups fresh spinach, chopped
- 1/2 cup crumbled feta cheese
- 2 cloves garlic, minced
- 1 tbsp olive oil
- 1/4 tsp salt
- 1/4 tsp black pepper

1. Preheat the oven to 400°F (200°C).

2. In a medium bowl, combine the chopped spinach, crumbled feta, minced garlic, 1 tsp of the olive oil, salt, and pepper. Mix well.

3. Using a sharp knife, cut a horizontal slit through the thickest part of each chicken breast to create a pocket, being careful not to cut all the way through.

4. Stuff each chicken breast with the spinach and feta mixture, dividing it evenly.

5. In a large oven-safe skillet or baking dish, heat the remaining 2 tsp of olive oil over medium-high heat.

6. Add the stuffed chicken breasts to the skillet or baking dish and sear for 2-3 minutes per side to lightly brown the outside.

7. Transfer the skillet or baking dish to the preheated oven and bake for 20-25 minutes, or until the chicken is cooked through and reaches an internal temperature of 165°F (75°C). Serve the stuffed chicken breasts immediately.

This recipe supports the MIND diet for seniors over 60 because it:
- Uses lean protein from chicken, which is recommended in the MIND diet.
- Includes spinach, which is a leafy green vegetable and part of the MIND diet's emphasis on plant-based foods.
- Features feta cheese, which provides healthy fats.
- Avoids processed ingredients and focuses on whole, unprocessed foods.

The MIND diet has been shown to help reduce the risk of cognitive decline and Alzheimer's disease in older adults. Enjoy this flavorful and nutritious stuffed chicken breast as part of a MIND diet-friendly meal plan.

How would you rate this dish?

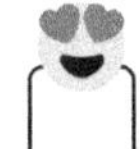 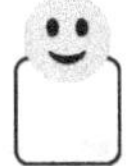  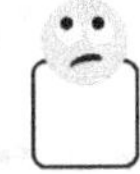 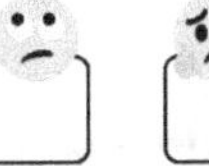

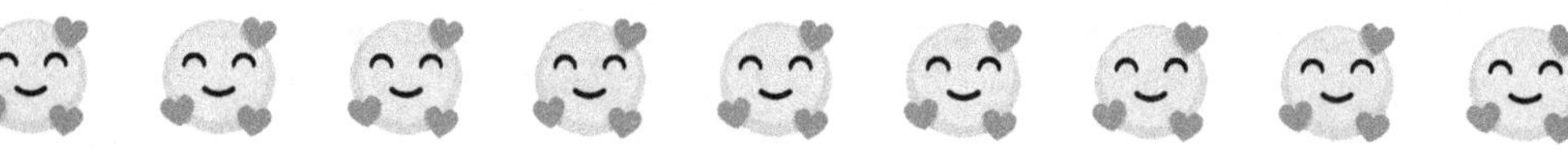

90. Turkey and vegetable kabobs

Let's do that and fill in the time here Prep Time :   Cook Time :   Servings :

Is this dish easy or difficult for you to make?

 ◯   ◯

Write 5 friends with whom you want to share this dish

____

____

____

____

____

INGREDIENTS

- 1 lb ground turkey
- 1 zucchini, cut into 1-inch pieces
- 1 red bell pepper, cut into 1-inch pieces
- 1 yellow onion, cut into 1-inch pieces
- 8 cherry tomatoes
- 2 tbsp olive oil
- 1 tsp dried oregano
- 1/2 tsp garlic powder
- 1/4 tsp salt
- 1/4 tsp black pepper

How would you rate this dish?

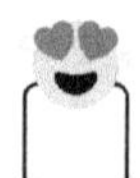 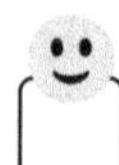 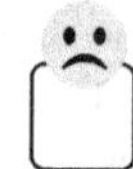 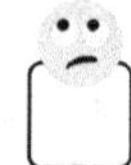 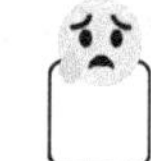

1. Preheat the grill or grill pan to medium-high heat.

2. In a large bowl, combine the ground turkey, zucchini, bell pepper, onion, and cherry tomatoes. Drizzle with the olive oil and sprinkle with the oregano, garlic powder, salt, and black pepper. Toss to coat the ingredients evenly.

3. Thread the turkey and vegetable pieces onto skewers, alternating the ingredients.

4. Grill the kabobs for 12-15 minutes, turning occasionally, until the turkey is cooked through and the vegetables are tender.

5. Serve the turkey and vegetable kabobs immediately.

This recipe supports the MIND diet for seniors over 60 because it:

- Uses lean protein from ground turkey, which is recommended in the MIND diet.

- Features a variety of vegetables, including zucchini, bell pepper, onion, and tomatoes, which are part of the MIND diet's emphasis on plant-based foods.

- Includes healthy fats from the olive oil.

- Avoids processed ingredients and focuses on whole, unprocessed foods.

The MIND diet has been shown to help reduce the risk of cognitive decline and Alzheimer's disease in older adults. Enjoy these flavorful and nutritious turkey and vegetable kabobs as part of a MIND diet-friendly meal plan.

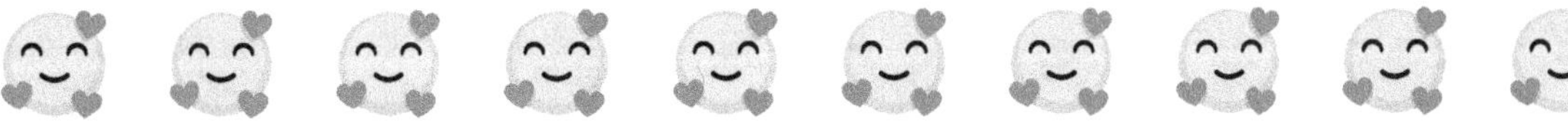

91. Wild rice pilaf with cranberries and almonds

 Prep Time :   Cook Time :   Servings :

Is this dish easy or difficult for you to make?

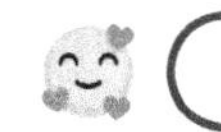 ◯   ◯

Write 5 ....
friends
with ....
whom
you ....
want to
share ....
this
dish ....

INGREDIENTS

- 1 cup uncooked wild rice
- 2 cups low-sodium chicken or vegetable broth
- 1/2 cup dried cranberries
- 1/4 cup sliced almonds
- 2 tbsp olive oil
- 1 shallot, minced
- 2 cloves garlic, minced
- 1 tsp dried thyme
- 1/4 tsp salt
- 1/4 tsp black pepper

1. In a medium saucepan, combine the wild rice and broth. Bring to a boil, then reduce heat to low, cover, and simmer for 45-50 minutes, or until the rice is tender and the liquid is absorbed.

2. In a small skillet, toast the sliced almonds over medium heat for 2-3 minutes, stirring frequently, until fragrant and lightly browned. Set aside.

3. In a large skillet or sauté pan, heat the olive oil over medium heat. Add the minced shallot and garlic, and cook for 2-3 minutes, until fragrant.

4. Fluff the cooked wild rice with a fork and add it to the skillet with the shallot and garlic. Stir in the dried cranberries, toasted almonds, thyme, salt, and black pepper. Cook for an additional 2-3 minutes, stirring occasionally, to allow the flavors to meld. Serve the wild rice pilaf warm.

This recipe supports the MIND diet for seniors over 60 because it:

- Uses whole grains from the wild rice, which is recommended in the MIND diet.

- Includes dried cranberries, which are a berry and part of the MIND diet's emphasis on plant-based foods.

- Features healthy fats from the almonds and olive oil.

- Avoids processed ingredients and focuses on whole, unprocessed foods.

The MIND diet has been shown to help reduce the risk of cognitive decline and Alzheimer's disease in older adults. Enjoy this flavorful and nutritious wild rice pilaf as part of a MIND diet-friendly meal plan.

How would you rate this dish?

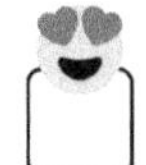 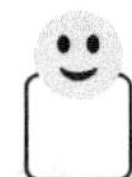 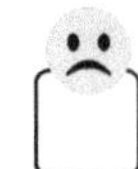 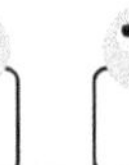 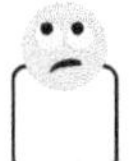 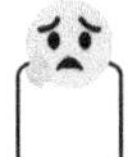

92. Barley risotto with mushrooms

 *Let's do that and fill in the time here* Prep Time :   Cook Time :   Servings :

Is this dish easy or difficult for you to make?

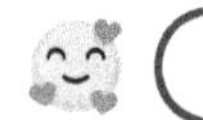 ◯   ◯

Write 5 friends with whom you want to share this dish

....
....
....
....
....

INGREDIENTS

- 1 cup pearl barley
- 4 cups low-sodium vegetable or chicken broth
- 2 tbsp olive oil
- 8 oz cremini or button mushrooms, sliced
- 1 onion, diced
- 3 cloves garlic, minced
- 1 tsp dried thyme
- 1/4 tsp salt
- 1/4 tsp black pepper
- 1/4 cup grated Parmesan cheese (optional)
- 2 tbsp chopped fresh parsley (for garnish)

How would you rate this dish?

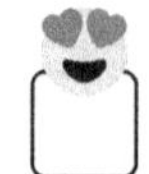 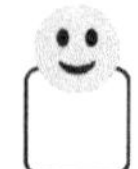 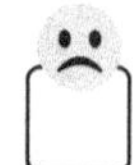 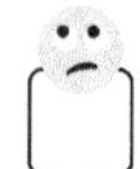 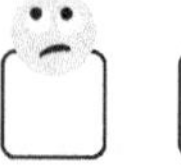 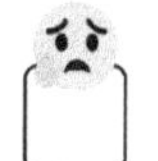

1. In a medium saucepan, bring the broth to a simmer over medium heat. Reduce heat to low and keep the broth warm.

2. In a large skillet, heat the olive oil over medium heat. Add the sliced mushrooms and cook for 5-7 minutes, stirring occasionally, until they are lightly browned.

3. Add the diced onion and minced garlic to the skillet. Cook for 2-3 minutes, until the onion is translucent.

4. Add the pearl barley to the skillet and stir to coat the grains with the oil. Cook for 2-3 minutes, stirring frequently, to toast the barley.

5. Ladle in 1/2 cup of the warm broth and stir constantly until the liquid is absorbed. Continue this process, adding 1/2 cup of broth at a time and stirring constantly, until the barley is tender and creamy, about 25-30 minutes total.

6. Stir in the dried thyme, salt, and black pepper. If desired, stir in the grated Parmesan cheese.

7. Serve the barley risotto warm, garnished with the chopped fresh parsley.

This recipe supports the MIND diet for seniors over 60 because it:

- Uses whole grains from the pearl barley, which is recommended in the MIND diet.

- Includes mushrooms, which are a vegetable and part of the MIND diet's emphasis on plant-based foods.

- Features healthy fats from the olive oil. Avoids processed ingredients and focuses on whole, unprocessed foods.

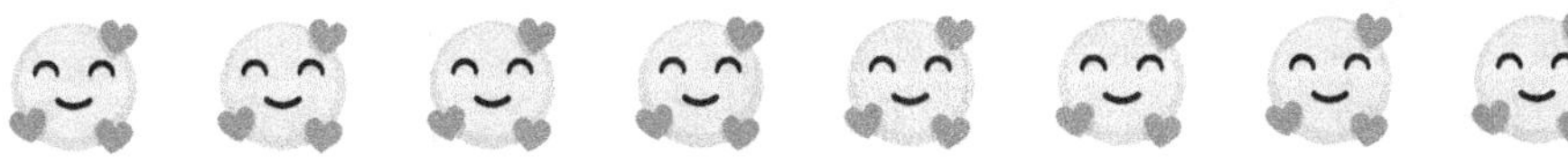

93. Quinoa and black bean bowl with cilantro lime dressing

Prep Time :   Cook Time :   Servings :

Is this dish easy or difficult for you to make?

 ◯   ◯

Write 5 friends with whom you want to share this dish ....

INGREDIENTS

For the Bowl:
- 1 cup uncooked quinoa, rinsed
- 1 (15 oz) can black beans, drained and rinsed
- 1 cup diced tomatoes
- 1 avocado, diced
- 1/2 cup diced red onion
- 1/4 cup chopped fresh cilantro

For the Dressing:
- 1/4 cup olive oil
- 2 tbsp lime juice
- 2 tbsp chopped fresh cilantro
- 1 clove garlic, minced
- 1/4 tsp salt
- 1/4 tsp black pepper

1. Cook the quinoa according to package instructions. Fluff with a fork and set aside.

2. In a large bowl, combine the cooked quinoa, black beans, diced tomatoes, avocado, red onion, and 1/4 cup chopped cilantro.

3. In a small bowl, whisk together the olive oil, lime juice, 2 tbsp chopped cilantro, minced garlic, salt, and black pepper to make the dressing.

4. Drizzle the cilantro lime dressing over the quinoa and black bean bowl and toss gently to coat.

5. Serve the quinoa and black bean bowl immediately.

This recipe supports the MIND diet for seniors over 60 because it:

- Uses whole grains from the quinoa, which is recommended in the MIND diet.

- Includes black beans, which are a legume and part of the MIND diet's emphasis on plant-based foods.

- Features healthy fats from the olive oil in the dressing.

- Includes vegetables like tomatoes, avocado, and onion, which are also key components of the MIND diet.

- Avoids processed ingredients and focuses on whole, unprocessed foods.

The MIND diet has been shown to help reduce the risk of cognitive decline and Alzheimer's disease in older adults. Enjoy this flavorful and nutritious quinoa and black bean bowl as part of a MIND diet-friendly meal plan.

How would you rate this dish?

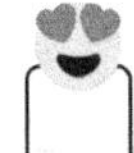 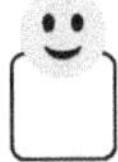 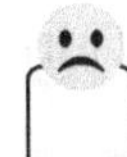 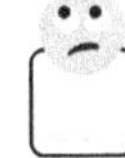 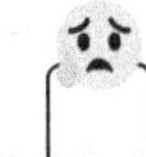

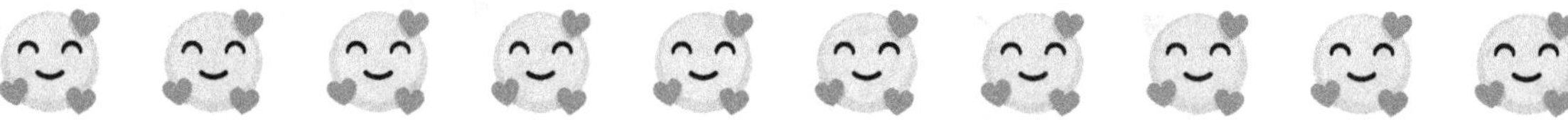

94. Bulgur wheat salad with pomegranate and mint

Let's do that and fill in the time here   Prep Time :   Cook Time :   Servings :

Is this dish easy or difficult for you to make?

 ○    ○

Write 5 friends with whom you want to share this dish

....

....

....

....

....

INGREDIENTS

- 1 cup uncooked bulgur wheat
- 1 1/2 cups boiling water
- 1 cup pomegranate arils
- 1/2 cup chopped fresh mint
- 1/4 cup chopped fresh parsley
- 1/4 cup olive oil
- 2 tbsp lemon juice
- 1 tsp honey
- 1/4 tsp salt
- 1/4 tsp black pepper

How would you rate this dish?

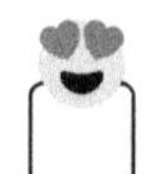 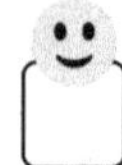 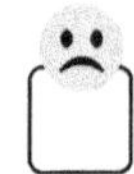 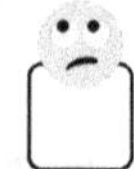 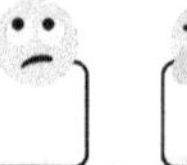 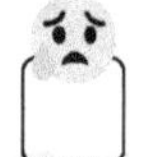

1. In a medium bowl, combine the uncooked bulgur wheat and boiling water. Cover and let sit for 15-20 minutes, until the bulgur is tender and the water is absorbed.

2. Fluff the cooked bulgur with a fork and transfer it to a large serving bowl.

3. Add the pomegranate arils, chopped mint, and chopped parsley to the bowl with the bulgur.

4. In a small bowl, whisk together the olive oil, lemon juice, honey, salt, and black pepper to make the dressing.

5. Pour the dressing over the bulgur salad and toss gently to coat. Serve the bulgur wheat salad chilled or at room temperature.

This recipe supports the MIND diet for seniors over 60 because it:

- Uses whole grains from the bulgur wheat, which is recommended in the MIND diet.

- Includes pomegranate arils, which are a fruit and part of the MIND diet's emphasis on plant-based foods.

- Features fresh herbs like mint and parsley, which are also key components of the MIND diet.

- Includes healthy fats from the olive oil in the dressing.
- Avoids processed ingredients and focuses on whole, unprocessed foods.

The MIND diet has been shown to help reduce the risk of cognitive decline and Alzheimer's disease in older adults. Enjoy this refreshing and nutritious bulgur wheat salad as part of a MIND diet-friendly meal plan.

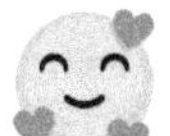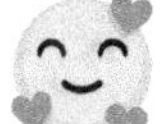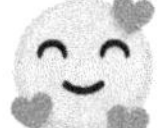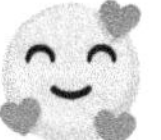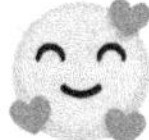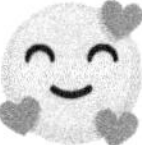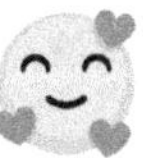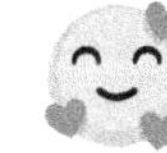

95. Farro and roasted vegetable bowl

Let's do that and fill in the time here   Prep Time :   Cook Time :   Servings :

Is this dish easy or difficult for you to make?

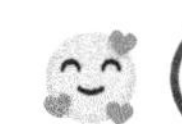 ◯   ◯

Write 5 friends with whom you want to share this dish
....
....
....
....
....

INGREDIENTS

- 1 cup uncooked farro
- 3 cups mixed vegetables (such as broccoli, cauliflower, bell peppers, zucchini), cut into 1-inch pieces
- 2 tbsp olive oil, divided
- 1/2 tsp salt, divided
- 1/4 tsp black pepper, divided
- 1 cup cherry tomatoes, halved
- 1/4 cup crumbled feta cheese
- 2 tbsp chopped fresh basil
- 2 tbsp balsamic vinegar

How would you rate this dish?

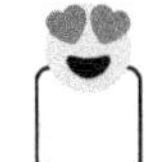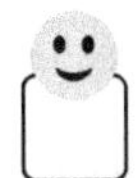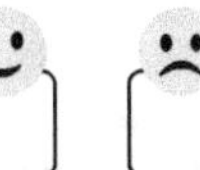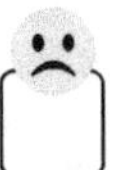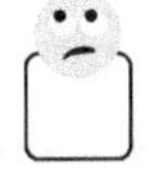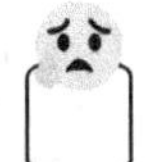

1. Preheat the oven to 400°F (200°C).

2. Cook the farro according to package instructions. Drain and set aside.

3. In a large bowl, toss the mixed vegetables with 1 tbsp of the olive oil, 1/4 tsp of the salt, and 1/8 tsp of the black pepper.

4. Spread the seasoned vegetables on a baking sheet and roast in the preheated oven for 20-25 minutes, or until tender and lightly browned.

5. In a large bowl, combine the cooked farro, roasted vegetables, cherry tomatoes, feta cheese, and chopped basil.

6. In a small bowl, whisk together the remaining 1 tbsp of olive oil, 1/4 tsp of salt, 1/8 tsp of black pepper, and the balsamic vinegar to make the dressing.

7. Drizzle the dressing over the farro and vegetable bowl and toss gently to coat. Serve the farro and roasted vegetable bowl warm or at room temperature.

This recipe supports the MIND diet for seniors over 60 because it:

- Uses whole grains from the farro, which is recommended in the MIND diet.
- Includes a variety of roasted vegetables, which are part of the MIND diet's emphasis on plant-based foods.
- Features healthy fats from the olive oil and feta cheese.
- Avoids processed ingredients and focuses on whole, unprocessed foods.

The MIND diet has been shown to help reduce the risk of cognitive decline and Alzheimer's disease in older adults. Enjoy this flavorful and nutritious farro and roasted vegetable bowl as part of a MIND diet-friendly meal plan.

96. Millet with roasted tomatoes and basil

Let's do that and fill in the time here   Prep Time :   Cook Time :   Servings :

Is this dish easy or difficult for you to make?

 ◯   ◯

Write 5 friends with whom you want to share this dish

....
....
....
....
....

INGREDIENTS

- 1 cup uncooked millet
- 2 cups low-sodium vegetable or chicken broth
- 1 lb cherry or grape tomatoes, halved
- 2 tbsp olive oil, divided
- 1/4 tsp salt
- 1/4 tsp black pepper
- 1/4 cup chopped fresh basil
- 2 tbsp balsamic glaze (optional)

How would you rate this dish?

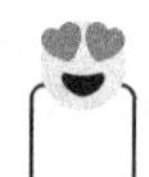 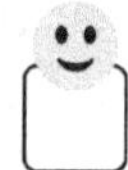 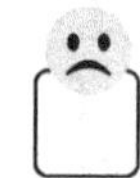 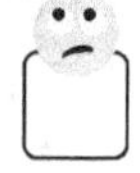  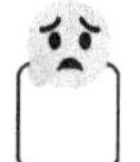

1. Preheat the oven to 400°F (200°C).

2. In a medium saucepan, combine the millet and broth. Bring to a boil, then reduce heat to low, cover, and simmer for 20-25 minutes, until the millet is tender and the liquid is absorbed.

3. While the millet is cooking, toss the halved tomatoes with 1 tbsp of the olive oil, salt, and black pepper on a baking sheet.

4. Roast the tomatoes in the preheated oven for 15-20 minutes, until they are softened and slightly charred.

5. In a large bowl, combine the cooked millet, roasted tomatoes, and the remaining 1 tbsp of olive oil. Toss to coat.

6. Stir in the chopped fresh basil. Serve the millet and roasted tomato mixture warm, drizzled with balsamic glaze if desired.

This recipe supports the MIND diet for seniors over 60 because it:

- Uses whole grains from the millet, which is recommended in the MIND diet.
- Includes roasted tomatoes, which are a vegetable and part of the MIND diet's emphasis on plant-based foods.
- Features fresh basil, which is also a key component of the MIND diet.
- Includes healthy fats from the olive oil.
- Avoids processed ingredients and focuses on whole, unprocessed foods.

The MIND diet has been shown to help reduce the risk of cognitive decline and Alzheimer's disease in older adults. Enjoy this flavorful and nutritious millet dish as part of a MIND diet-friendly meal plan.

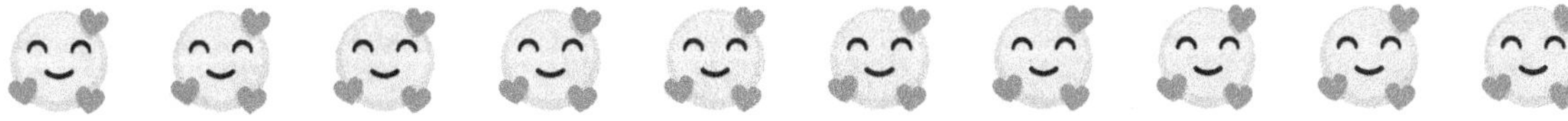

97. Brown rice stir-fry with tofu and vegetables

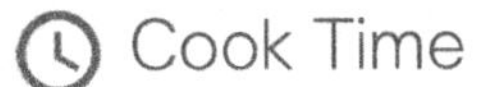 Prep Time :   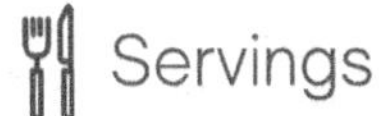 Cook Time :   Servings :

Is this dish easy or difficult for you to make?

 ◯   ◯

Write 5 friends with whom you want to share this dish

....

....

....

....

....

INGREDIENTS

- 1 cup uncooked brown rice
- 1 block (14 oz) extra-firm tofu, cubed
- 2 tbsp sesame oil, divided
- 1 cup sliced mushrooms
- 1 cup broccoli florets
- 1 red bell pepper, sliced
- 1 cup snow peas or snap peas
- 3 cloves garlic, minced
- 1 tbsp grated fresh ginger
- 2 tbsp low-sodium soy sauce
- 1 tbsp rice vinegar
- 1 tsp honey
- 1/4 tsp red pepper flakes (optional)
- 2 tbsp chopped fresh cilantro (for garnish)

1. Cook the brown rice according to package instructions. Set aside.

2. In a large skillet or wok, heat 1 tbsp of the sesame oil over medium-high heat. Add the cubed tofu and cook, stirring occasionally, until lightly browned on all sides, about 5-7 minutes. Transfer the tofu to a plate and set aside.

3. In the same skillet, heat the remaining 1 tbsp of sesame oil over medium-high heat. Add the mushrooms, broccoli, bell pepper, and snow peas. Stir-fry for 5-7 minutes, until the vegetables are tender-crisp.

4. Add the minced garlic and grated ginger to the skillet and cook for 1 minute, until fragrant.

5. Return the cooked tofu to the skillet. Add the cooked brown rice, soy sauce, rice vinegar, and honey. Toss everything together and cook for 2-3 minutes, until heated through.

6. Remove from heat and stir in the red pepper flakes, if using. Serve the brown rice stir-fry warm, garnished with chopped fresh cilantro.

This recipe supports the MIND diet for seniors over 60 because it:

- Uses whole grains from the brown rice, which is recommended in the MIND diet.
- Includes tofu, which is a plant-based protein and part of the MIND diet's emphasis on plant-based foods.
- Features a variety of vegetables like mushrooms, broccoli, bell pepper, and snow peas, which are also key components of the MIND diet.
- Includes healthy fats from the sesame oil.
- Avoids processed ingredients and focuses on whole, unprocessed foods.

How would you rate this dish?

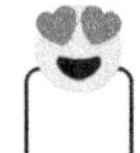 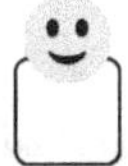 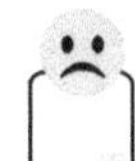 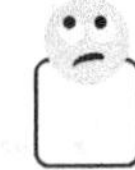 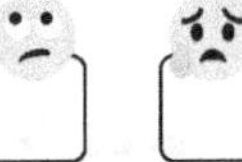 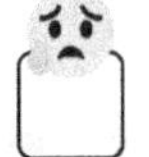

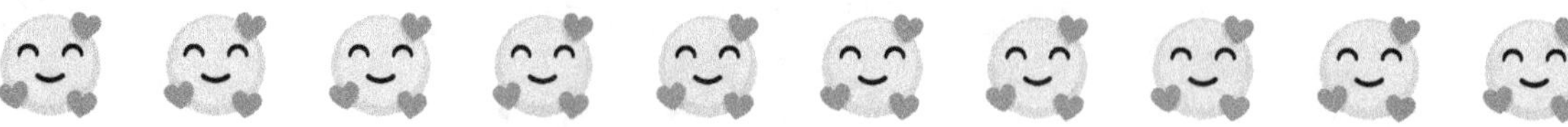

98. Couscous with grilled vegetables and chickpeas

 Prep Time :   Cook Time :   Servings :

Is this dish easy or difficult for you to make?

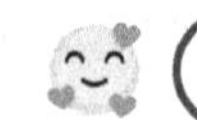 ◯   ◯

Write 5 friends with whom you want to share this dish

....

....

....

....

INGREDIENTS

- 1 cup uncooked whole wheat couscous
- 1 1/4 cups low-sodium vegetable broth
- 1 zucchini, sliced into 1/2-inch rounds
- 1 red bell pepper, cut into 1-inch pieces
- 1 red onion, cut into 1-inch wedges
- 2 tbsp olive oil, divided
- 1/4 tsp salt
- 1/4 tsp black pepper
- 1 (15 oz) can chickpeas, drained and rinsed
- 2 tbsp chopped fresh parsley
- 1 tbsp lemon juice

How would you rate this dish?

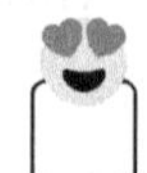 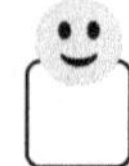 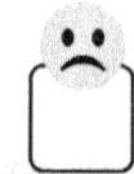 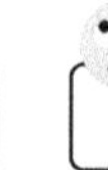 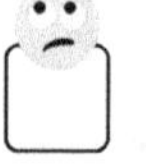 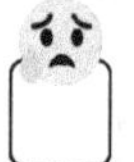

1. Prepare the couscous according to package instructions, using the vegetable broth instead of water. Fluff with a fork and set aside.

2. Preheat the grill or grill pan to medium-high heat.

3. In a large bowl, toss the zucchini, bell pepper, and onion with 1 tbsp of the olive oil, salt, and black pepper.

4. Grill the vegetables for 8-10 minutes, turning occasionally, until they are tender and lightly charred.

5. In a large bowl, combine the cooked couscous, grilled vegetables, chickpeas, 1 tbsp of olive oil, chopped parsley, and lemon juice. Toss gently to mix.

6. Serve the couscous and vegetable salad warm or at room temperature.

This recipe supports the MIND diet for seniors over 60 because it:

- Uses whole grains from the whole wheat couscous, which is recommended in the MIND diet.
- Includes a variety of grilled vegetables like zucchini, bell pepper, and onion, which are part of the MIND diet's emphasis on plant-based foods.
- Features chickpeas, which are a legume and also a key component of the MIND diet.
- Includes healthy fats from the olive oil.
- Avoids processed ingredients and focuses on whole, unprocessed foods.

The MIND diet has been shown to help reduce the risk of cognitive decline and Alzheimer's disease in older adults. Enjoy this flavorful and nutritious couscous salad as part of a MIND diet-friendly meal plan.

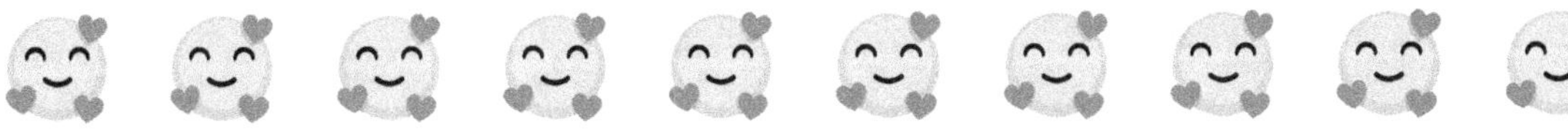

99. Polenta with sautéed spinach and mushrooms

Prep Time :   Cook Time :   Servings :

Is this dish easy or difficult for you to make?

 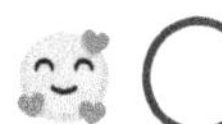

Write 5 friends with whom you want to share this dish

....

....

....

....

....

INGREDIENTS

- 1 cup uncooked polenta
- 4 cups low-sodium vegetable or chicken broth
- 1/4 tsp salt
- 1 tbsp olive oil
- 8 oz cremini or button mushrooms, sliced
- 3 cloves garlic, minced
- 5 oz baby spinach
- 1/4 cup grated Parmesan cheese (optional)
- 1 tbsp chopped fresh basil (for garnish)

How would you rate this dish?

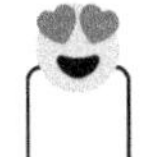 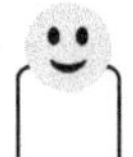  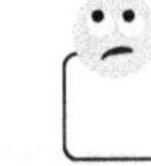 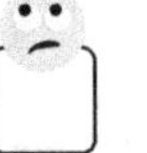 

1. In a medium saucepan, bring the broth to a boil over high heat. Slowly whisk in the polenta and salt. Reduce heat to low and cook, stirring frequently, for 15-20 minutes, until the polenta is thick and creamy.

2. In a large skillet, heat the olive oil over medium-high heat. Add the sliced mushrooms and cook for 5-7 minutes, until they are lightly browned.

3. Add the minced garlic to the skillet and cook for 1 minute, until fragrant.

4. Add the baby spinach to the skillet and cook for 2-3 minutes, stirring frequently, until the spinach is wilted.

5. Spoon the cooked polenta into serving bowls. Top with the sautéed spinach and mushrooms.

6. If desired, sprinkle the polenta and vegetables with grated Parmesan cheese. Garnish with chopped fresh basil before serving.

This recipe supports the MIND diet for seniors over 60 because it:

- Uses whole grains from the polenta, which is recommended in the MIND diet.
- Includes spinach and mushrooms, which are vegetables and part of the MIND diet's emphasis on plant-based foods.
- Features healthy fats from the olive oil.
- Includes optional Parmesan cheese, which provides some dairy.
- Avoids processed ingredients and focuses on whole, unprocessed foods.

The MIND diet has been shown to help reduce the risk of cognitive decline and Alzheimer's disease in older adults. Enjoy this flavorful and nutritious polenta dish as part of a MIND diet-friendly meal plan.

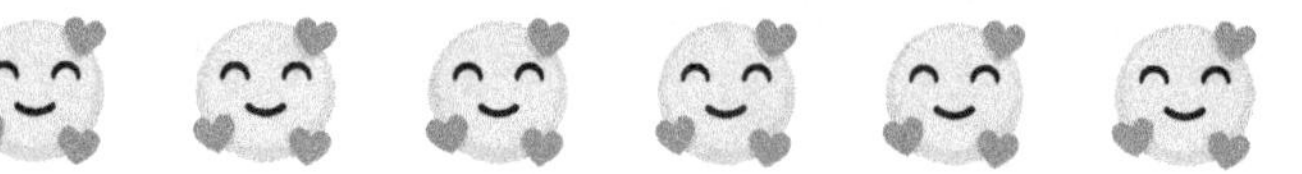

100. Wild rice and lentil casserole

Prep Time :   Cook Time :   Servings :

Is this dish easy or difficult for you to make?

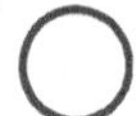 ◯   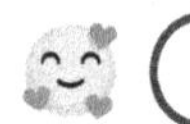 ◯

Write 5 friends with whom you want to share this dish ....

INGREDIENTS

- 1 cup uncooked wild rice
- 1 cup dry brown or green lentils, rinsed
- 4 cups vegetable or chicken broth
- 1 onion, diced
- 3 cloves garlic, minced
- 2 carrots, peeled and diced
- 2 celery stalks, diced
- 1 cup sliced mushrooms
- 1 tsp dried thyme
- 1 tsp dried rosemary
- Salt and pepper to taste
- 1/2 cup shredded cheddar cheese (optional)

1. Preheat oven to 375°F.

2. In a large pot, combine the wild rice, lentils, and broth. Bring to a boil, then reduce heat and simmer for 30-35 minutes, until rice and lentils are tender. Drain any excess liquid.

3. In a large skillet, sauté the onion, garlic, carrots, celery, and mushrooms in a bit of olive oil until softened, about 5-7 minutes.

4. Transfer the cooked rice and lentils to a 9x13 baking dish. Stir in the sautéed vegetables, thyme, rosemary, salt, and pepper.

5. If using, sprinkle the shredded cheddar cheese over the top.

6. Bake for 20-25 minutes, until heated through and cheese is melted.

7. Serve hot. This casserole makes a great main dish or side.

This wild rice and lentil casserole is a nutritious and comforting meal that is perfect for seniors over 60. The combination of whole grains, plant-based protein, and vegetables provides a wealth of fiber, vitamins, minerals, and antioxidants to support overall health. Enjoy!

How would you rate this dish?

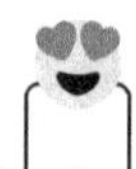 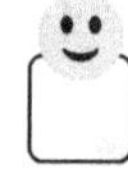 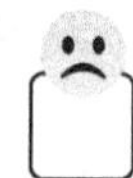 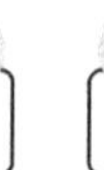 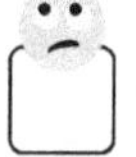 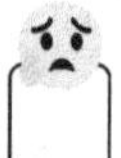

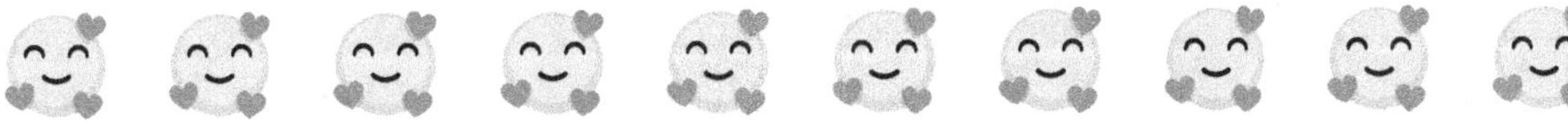

101. Berry parfait with Greek yogurt and honey

Prep Time :   Cook Time :   Servings :

Is this dish easy or difficult for you to make?

 ○   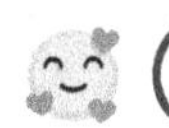 ○

Write 5 friends with whom you want to share this dish

....
....
....
....
....

INGREDIENTS

- 2 cups plain Greek yogurt
- 1 cup mixed fresh berries (such as blueberries, raspberries, and blackberries)
- 2-3 tablespoons honey
- 1/4 cup granola (optional)

1. In a parfait glass or small bowl, layer the ingredients in the following order:
   - 1/4 cup Greek yogurt
   - 1/4 cup mixed berries
   - 1 teaspoon honey
   - Repeat the layers until you reach the top of the glass.

2. If using granola, sprinkle a tablespoon or two over the top of the parfait.

3. Serve chilled or at room temperature.

This berry parfait is a wonderful and healthy treat for seniors over 60 for several reasons:

1. Greek yogurt is an excellent source of protein, calcium, and probiotics, which are important for bone health and gut health.

2. Berries are packed with antioxidants, fiber, and vitamins that can help support cognitive function, immune health, and reduce inflammation.

3. Honey provides a natural sweetener that is rich in antioxidants and has been shown to have anti-inflammatory properties.

4. The combination of the creamy yogurt, sweet berries, and honey creates a delicious and satisfying dessert or snack.

5. The parfait can be easily customized with different types of berries or other fresh fruit, making it a versatile and nutritious option.

Enjoy this berry parfait as a healthy and delicious way to incorporate more nutrient-dense foods into your diet. It's a great option for seniors looking to support their overall health and well-being.

How would you rate this dish?

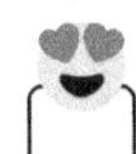 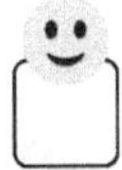  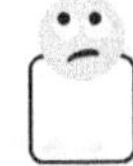 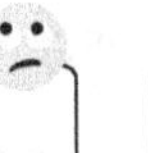 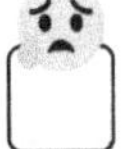

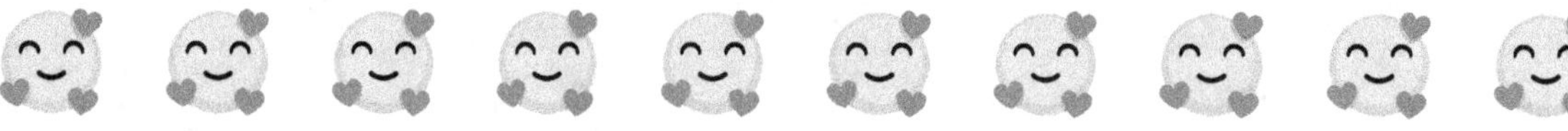

102. Baked apples with cinnamon and walnuts

Let's do that and fill in the time here ✓ Prep Time :   🕐 Cook Time :   🍴 Servings :

Is this dish easy or difficult for you to make?

 ◯    ◯

Write 5 friends with whom you want to share this dish

....
....
....
....
....

INGREDIENTS

- 4 medium-sized apples (such as Honeycrisp or Gala)
- 1/4 cup chopped walnuts
- 2 tbsp honey
- 1 tsp ground cinnamon
- 1/4 tsp ground nutmeg
- 2 tbsp water

1. Preheat the oven to 375°F (190°C).

2. Core the apples, leaving a small well in the center of each one. Place the apples in a baking dish.

3. In a small bowl, mix together the chopped walnuts, honey, cinnamon, and nutmeg.

4. Spoon the walnut mixture into the center of each apple, packing it in gently.

5. Pour the water into the bottom of the baking dish.

6. Bake the apples for 30-35 minutes, or until they are tender when pierced with a fork.

7. Serve the baked apples warm, with the juices from the baking dish spooned over the top.

This recipe supports the MIND diet for seniors over 60 because it:

- Uses apples, which are a fruit and part of the MIND diet's emphasis on plant-based foods.

- Includes walnuts, which provide healthy fats and are a key component of the MIND diet.

- Features cinnamon and nutmeg, which are spices that can provide additional health benefits.

- Uses honey as a natural sweetener. Avoids processed ingredients and focuses on whole, unprocessed foods.

The MIND diet has been shown to help reduce the risk of cognitive decline and Alzheimer's disease in older adults. These baked apples with cinnamon and walnuts make for a delicious and nutritious dessert or snack that aligns with the MIND diet guidelines.

How would you rate this dish?

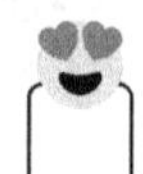 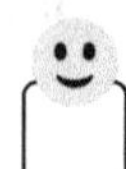 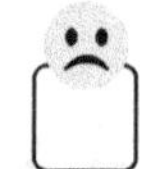 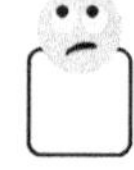 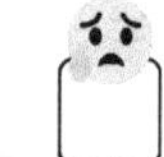

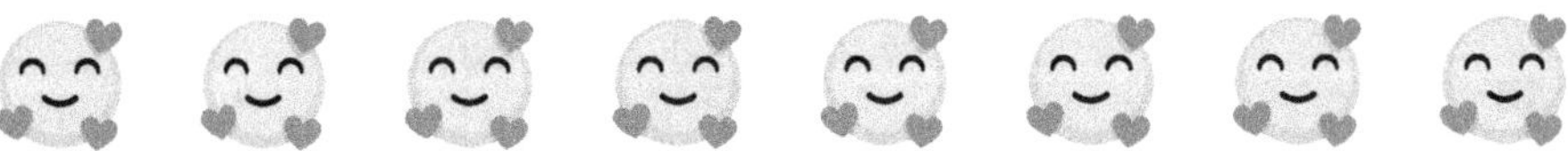

103. Dark chocolate-dipped strawberries

 *Let's do that and fill in the time here* Prep Time :   Cook Time :   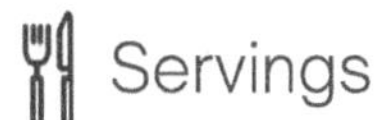 Servings :

Is this dish easy or difficult for you to make?

Write 5 friends with whom you want to share this dish ....

INGREDIENTS

- 1 lb fresh strawberries, washed and patted dry
- 4 oz dark chocolate (at least 70% cacao), chopped

1. Line a baking sheet with parchment paper or a silicone baking mat.

2. In a double boiler or a heatproof bowl set over a saucepan of simmering water, melt the chopped dark chocolate, stirring occasionally, until smooth.

3. Holding them by the stem, dip each strawberry into the melted chocolate, coating about three-quarters of the berry.

4. Gently tap off any excess chocolate and place the dipped strawberries on the prepared baking sheet.

5. Refrigerate the chocolate-dipped strawberries for at least 30 minutes, or until the chocolate has set.

6. Serve the dark chocolate-dipped strawberries chilled.

This recipe supports the MIND diet for seniors over 60 because it:

- Uses dark chocolate, which is rich in antioxidants and a key component of the MIND diet.

- Includes fresh strawberries, which are a fruit and part of the MIND diet's emphasis on plant-based foods.

- Avoids processed ingredients and focuses on whole, unprocessed foods.

The MIND diet has been shown to help reduce the risk of cognitive decline and Alzheimer's disease in older adults. These dark chocolate-dipped strawberries provide a delicious and nutritious treat that aligns with the MIND diet guidelines.

How would you rate this dish?

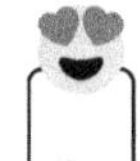 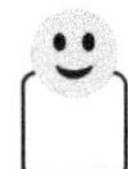 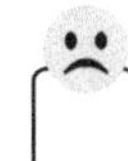 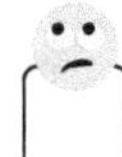 

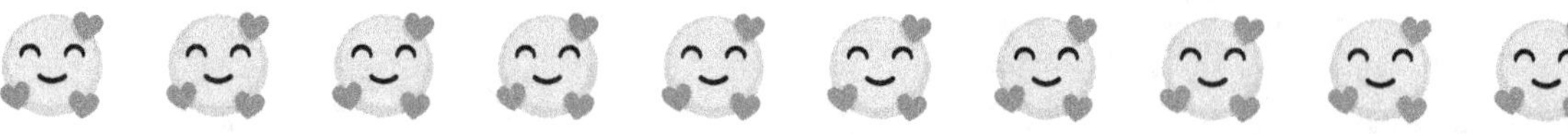

104. Chia seed pudding with mango puree

Let's do that and fill in the time here

Is this dish easy or difficult for you to make?

 ◯    ◯

Write 5 friends with whom you want to share this dish

....

....

....

....

....

INGREDIENTS

- 1/4 cup chia seeds
- 1 cup unsweetened almond milk
- 2 tbsp honey
- 1 tsp vanilla extract
- 1 ripe mango, peeled and diced
- 1 tbsp water

1. In a medium bowl, whisk together the chia seeds, almond milk, honey, and vanilla extract. Cover and refrigerate for at least 2 hours, or up to 24 hours, stirring occasionally, until thickened.

2. In a blender or food processor, puree the diced mango with 1 tbsp of water until smooth.

3. Divide the chia seed pudding into 4 serving bowls or glasses.

4. Top each serving of chia pudding with a dollop of the mango puree.

5. Serve chilled.

This recipe supports the MIND diet for seniors over 60 because it:

- Uses chia seeds, which are a source of healthy fats, fiber, and protein.

- Includes mango, which is a fruit and part of the MIND diet's emphasis on plant-based foods.

- Features unsweetened almond milk, which provides a dairy-free, low-sugar option.

- Uses honey as a natural sweetener. Avoids processed ingredients and focuses on whole, unprocessed foods.

The MIND diet has been shown to help reduce the risk of cognitive decline and Alzheimer's disease in older adults. This refreshing and nutritious chia seed pudding with mango puree makes for a delightful and MIND diet-friendly snack or dessert.

How would you rate this dish?

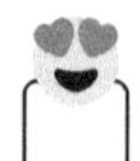 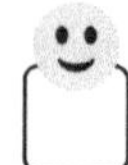 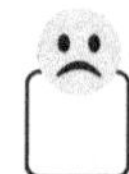  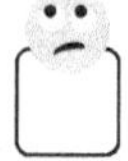 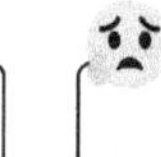

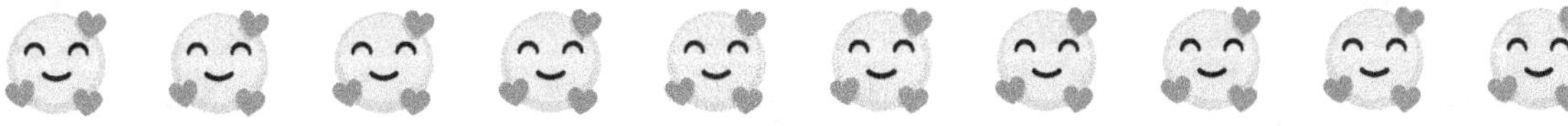

105. Oatmeal cookies with raisins and walnuts

Prep Time :   Cook Time :   Servings :

Is this dish easy or difficult for you to make?

 ◯   ◯

Write 5 friends with whom you want to share this dish ....

INGREDIENTS

- 1 cup whole wheat flour
- 1 tsp baking soda
- 1/2 tsp ground cinnamon
- 1/4 tsp salt
- 1 cup old-fashioned oats
- 1/2 cup unsalted butter, softened
- 1/2 cup brown sugar
- 1 egg
- 1 tsp vanilla extract
- 1/2 cup raisins
- 1/2 cup chopped walnuts

How would you rate this dish?

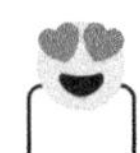 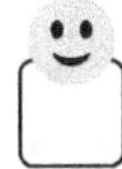 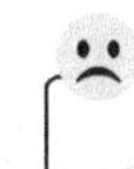 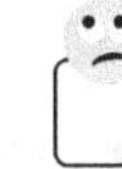 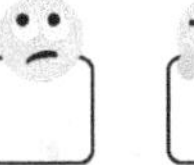 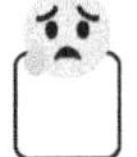

1. Preheat the oven to 350°F (175°C). Line a baking sheet with parchment paper.

2. In a medium bowl, whisk together the whole wheat flour, baking soda, cinnamon, and salt. Stir in the old-fashioned oats.

3. In a large bowl, beat the softened butter and brown sugar together until light and fluffy. Beat in the egg and vanilla extract.

4. Gradually add the dry ingredients to the wet ingredients, mixing just until combined. Fold in the raisins and chopped walnuts.

5. Scoop rounded tablespoons of dough onto the prepared baking sheet, spacing them about 2 inches apart.

6. Bake for 10-12 minutes, or until the cookies are lightly golden around the edges.

7. Allow the cookies to cool on the baking sheet for 5 minutes before transferring to a wire rack to cool completely.

This recipe supports the MIND diet for seniors over 60 because it:

- Uses whole grains from the whole wheat flour and old-fashioned oats, which are recommended in the MIND diet.
- Includes raisins, which are a fruit and part of the MIND diet's emphasis on plant-based foods.
- Features walnuts, which provide healthy fats and are also a key component of the MIND diet.
- Avoids processed ingredients and uses natural sweeteners like brown sugar.

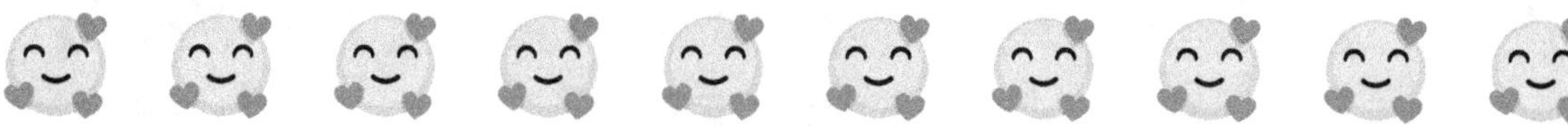

106. Banana and almond butter bites

  Prep Time :   Cook Time :   Servings :

Is this dish easy or difficult for you to make?

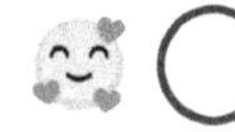 ◯   ◯

Write 5 ....
friends
with ....
whom
you ....
want to
share ....
this
dish ....

INGREDIENTS

- 2 ripe bananas, sliced into 1/2-inch rounds
- 1/4 cup creamy almond butter
- 2 tbsp chopped roasted unsalted almonds

1. Line a baking sheet with parchment paper.

2. Spread a small amount of almond butter (about 1 tsp) onto each banana slice.

3. Sprinkle the chopped almonds over the almond butter-topped banana slices.

4. Place the banana bites on the prepared baking sheet and freeze for at least 2 hours, or until firm.

5. Once frozen, transfer the banana bites to an airtight container or resealable plastic bag and store in the freezer until ready to serve.

This recipe supports the MIND diet for seniors over 60 because it:

- Uses bananas, which are a fruit and part of the MIND diet's emphasis on plant-based foods.

- Includes almond butter, which provides healthy fats and is a key component of the MIND diet.

- Features chopped roasted almonds, which are also a source of healthy fats and part of the MIND diet.

- Avoids processed ingredients and focuses on whole, unprocessed foods.

The MIND diet has been shown to help reduce the risk of cognitive decline and Alzheimer's disease in older adults. These frozen banana and almond butter bites make for a delicious and nutritious snack or dessert that aligns with the MIND diet guidelines.

How would you rate this dish?

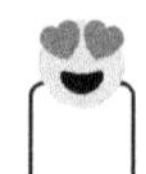 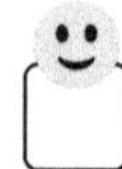 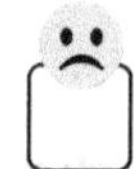 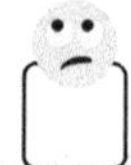 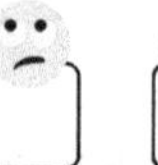 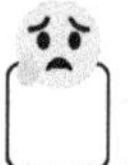

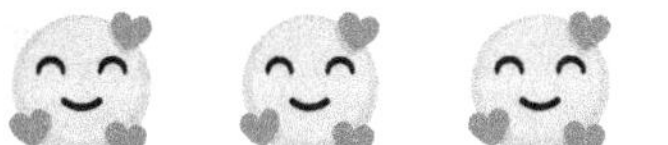

107. Whole-grain blueberry muffins

Let's do that and fill in the time here 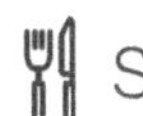 Prep Time :   Cook Time :   Servings :

Is this dish easy or difficult for you to make?

 ○   ◌ ○

Write 5 friends with whom you want to share this dish

....
....
....
....
....

INGREDIENTS

- 1 cup whole wheat flour
- 1 cup old-fashioned oats
- 1 tsp baking powder
- 1/2 tsp baking soda
- 1/4 tsp salt
- 1 egg
- 1/2 cup plain Greek yogurt
- 1/3 cup honey
- 2 tbsp unsweetened applesauce
- 1 tsp vanilla extract
- 1 cup fresh or frozen blueberries

How would you rate this dish?

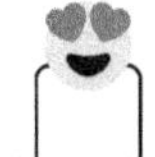 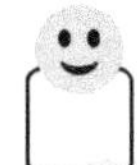 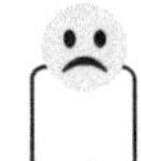 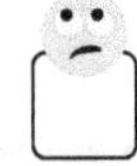 

1. Preheat the oven to 375°F (190°C). Grease a 12-cup muffin tin or line with paper liners.

2. In a medium bowl, whisk together the whole wheat flour, oats, baking powder, baking soda, and salt.

3. In a separate bowl, beat the egg. Then stir in the Greek yogurt, honey, applesauce, and vanilla extract until well combined.

4. Gently fold the wet ingredients into the dry ingredients, being careful not to overmix. Fold in the blueberries.

5. Spoon the batter evenly into the prepared muffin cups, filling them about 3/4 full.

6. Bake for 18-20 minutes, or until a toothpick inserted into the center comes out clean.

7. Allow the muffins to cool in the tin for 5 minutes before transferring to a wire rack to cool completely.

This recipe supports the MIND diet for seniors over 60 because it:

- Uses whole grains from the whole wheat flour and oats, which are recommended in the MIND diet.
- Includes blueberries, which are a fruit and part of the MIND diet's emphasis on plant-based foods.
- Features healthy fats and proteins from the Greek yogurt.
- Avoids processed ingredients and uses natural sweeteners like honey.

The MIND diet has been shown to help reduce the risk of cognitive decline and Alzheimer's disease in older adults. Enjoy these wholesome and delicious blueberry muffins as a nutritious snack or breakfast option as part of a MIND diet-friendly meal plan.

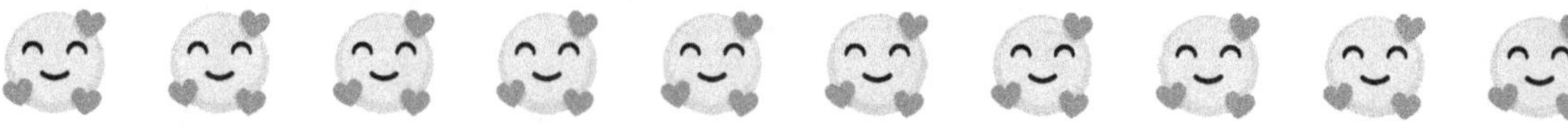

108. Greek yogurt with pomegranate seeds and honey

Prep Time :   Cook Time :   Servings :

Is this dish easy or difficult for you to make?

 ◯   ◯

Write 5 ....
friends
with ....
whom
you ....
want to
share ....
this
dish ....

INGREDIENTS

- 1 cup plain Greek yogurt
- 1/2 cup pomegranate seeds
- 2 tbsp honey

How would you rate this dish?

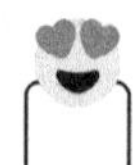 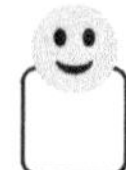 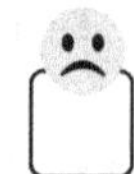  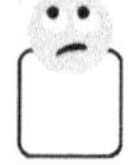 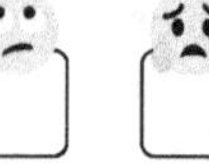

1. Scoop the Greek yogurt into a serving bowl or individual bowls.

2. Sprinkle the pomegranate seeds over the yogurt.

3. Drizzle the honey over the top. Serve immediately.

This recipe supports the MIND diet for seniors over 60 because it:

- Uses dairy from the Greek yogurt, which is recommended in the MIND diet.

- Includes pomegranate seeds, which are a fruit and part of the MIND diet's emphasis on plant-based foods.

- Features honey, which is a natural sweetener.

- Avoids processed ingredients and focuses on whole, unprocessed foods.

The MIND diet has been shown to help reduce the risk of cognitive decline and Alzheimer's disease in older adults. This simple yet delicious Greek yogurt parfait provides a nutritious and satisfying snack or dessert that aligns with the MIND diet guidelines.

Some additional tips:

- Choose plain, unsweetened Greek yogurt to minimize added sugars.
- Look for pomegranate seeds that are in season for maximum freshness and flavor.
- Use a high-quality, raw honey if possible for added health benefits.
- You can also try adding a sprinkle of chopped nuts, such as almonds or walnuts, for extra crunch and healthy fats

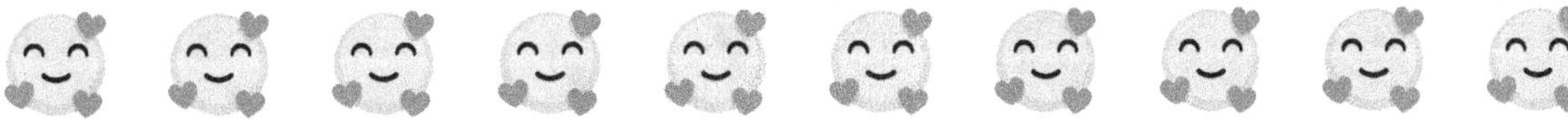

109. Homemade granola bars with nuts and dried fruit

Prep Time :   Cook Time :   Servings :

Is this dish easy or difficult for you to make?

 ◯   ◯

Write 5 ....
friends
with   ....
whom
you   ....
want to
share   ....
this
dish   ....

INGREDIENTS

- 2 cups old-fashioned oats
- 1/2 cup chopped walnuts
- 1/2 cup chopped almonds
- 1/4 cup ground flaxseed
- 1/4 cup honey
- 1/4 cup unsweetened applesauce
- 1 tsp vanilla extract
- 1/4 tsp salt
- 1/2 cup chopped dried apricots or cranberries

1. Preheat the oven to 325°F (165°C). Line an 8x8-inch baking pan with parchment paper, leaving some overhang on the sides for easy removal.

2. In a large bowl, combine the old-fashioned oats, chopped walnuts, chopped almonds, and ground flaxseed.

3. In a separate bowl, whisk together the honey, unsweetened applesauce, vanilla extract, and salt.

4. Pour the wet ingredients into the dry ingredients and stir until well combined. Fold in the chopped dried fruit.

5. Press the granola bar mixture firmly into the prepared baking pan, using your hands or the back of a spoon to compact it.

6. Bake for 20-25 minutes, or until the edges are lightly golden.

7. Allow the granola bars to cool completely in the pan, then use the parchment paper to lift them out. Cut into 12 bars.

8. Store the granola bars in an airtight container at room temperature for up to 1 week.

This recipe supports the MIND diet for seniors over 60 because it:

- Uses whole grains from the old-fashioned oats, which are recommended in the MIND diet.
- Includes nuts like walnuts and almonds, which provide healthy fats and are a key component of the MIND diet.
- Features dried fruit, which is a plant-based food and part of the MIND diet's emphasis on fruits and vegetables.

How would you rate this dish?

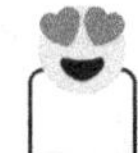 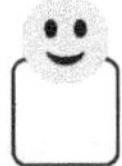  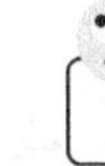 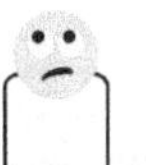 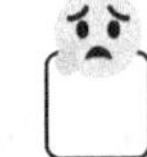

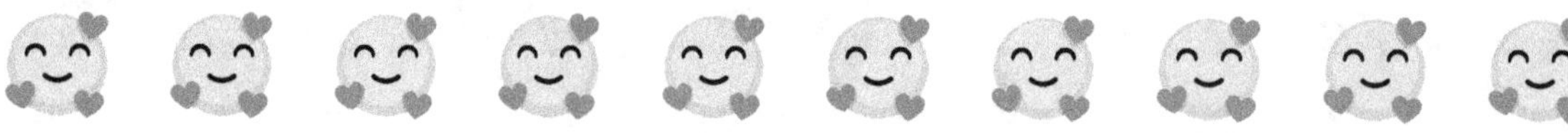

110. Baked pears with a sprinkle of cinnamon

 Prep Time :   Cook Time :   Servings :

Is this dish easy or difficult for you to make?

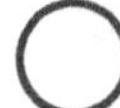 ◯   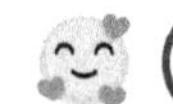 ◯

Write 5 friends with whom you want to share this dish

....

....

....

....

....

INGREDIENTS

- 4 ripe but firm pears, halved and cored
- 2 tbsp unsalted butter, melted
- 2 tsp ground cinnamon
- 2 tbsp brown sugar

1. Preheat your oven to 375°F (190°C).

2. Arrange the pear halves, cut-side up, in a baking dish or on a rimmed baking sheet.

3. Brush the pear halves with the melted butter, making sure to coat the tops and sides.

4. Sprinkle the cinnamon evenly over the pears, followed by the brown sugar.

5. Bake for 20-25 minutes, or until the pears are tender when pierced with a fork. The sugar should have caramelized slightly.

6. Serve the baked pears warm, either on their own or with a scoop of vanilla ice cream or a dollop of whipped cream, if desired.

The combination of the sweet, juicy pears and the warm cinnamon-sugar topping makes for a simple yet delicious dessert. Enjoy!

How would you rate this dish?

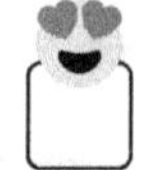 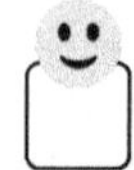  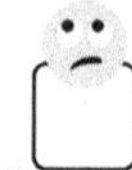 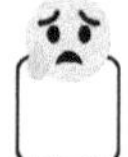

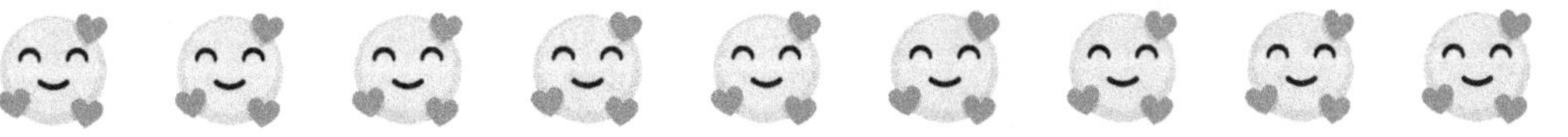

111. Green smoothie with kale, apple, and ginger

 Prep Time : 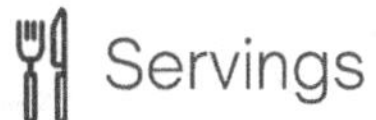 Cook Time : Servings :

Is this dish easy or difficult for you to make?

○   ○

Write 5 ....
friends
with ....
whom
you ....
want to
share ....
this
dish ....

INGREDIENTS

- 1 cup packed kale leaves, stems removed
- 1 medium apple, cored and chopped
- 1-inch piece of fresh ginger, peeled and grated
- 1 cup unsweetened almond milk
- 1 tbsp honey (optional)
- 1 cup ice cubes

1. Add the kale, apple, grated ginger, almond milk, and honey (if using) to a high-speed blender.

2. Blend on high speed until the mixture is smooth and creamy, about 1-2 minutes.

3. Add the ice cubes and blend again until the smoothie is thick and chilled, about 30 seconds to 1 minute.

4. Pour the green smoothie into a glass and enjoy immediately.

This smoothie is a great way to incorporate the key components of the MIND diet, which is designed to support brain health and cognitive function in older adults:

- Kale is a leafy green vegetable that is rich in antioxidants, vitamins, and minerals.

- Apples are a good source of fiber, vitamin C, and flavonoids, which have been linked to improved cognitive function.

- Ginger is a potent anti-inflammatory and has been shown to have neuroprotective effects.

- Almond milk is a dairy-free, low-calorie option that provides healthy fats and minerals.

The MIND diet emphasizes the consumption of these types of nutrient-dense, plant-based foods to help reduce the risk of age-related cognitive decline and dementia. Enjoy this smoothie as a healthy and delicious way to support your brain health!

How would you rate this dish?

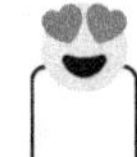 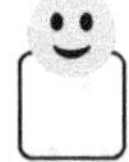 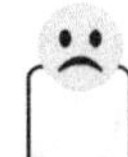 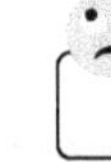 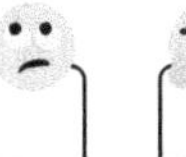

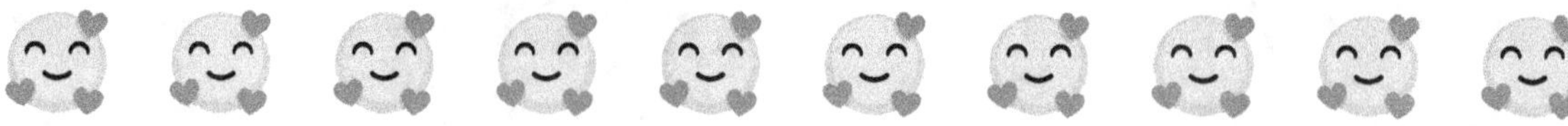

112. Berry and spinach smoothie with almond milk

Let's do that and fill in the time here Prep Time :   Cook Time :   Servings :

Is this dish easy or difficult for you to make?

 ○   ○

Write 5 friends with whom you want to share this dish

....

....

....

....

....

INGREDIENTS

- 1 cup fresh or frozen mixed berries (such as blueberries, raspberries, and blackberries)
- 1 cup packed fresh spinach leaves
- 1 cup unsweetened almond milk
- 1 tbsp honey (optional)
- 1 cup ice cubes

1. Add the mixed berries, spinach, almond milk, and honey (if using) to a high-speed blender.

2. Blend on high speed until the mixture is smooth and creamy, about 1-2 minutes.

3. Add the ice cubes and blend again until the smoothie is thick and chilled, about 30 seconds to 1 minute.

4. Pour the smoothie into a glass and enjoy immediately.

This smoothie is a great way to incorporate a variety of nutrient-dense ingredients that can support overall health and well-being for seniors over 60:

- Berries are rich in antioxidants, fiber, and vitamins that can help reduce inflammation and support cognitive function.

- Spinach is a leafy green vegetable that is packed with vitamins, minerals, and plant-based compounds that can support eye health, bone health, and immune function.

- Almond milk is a dairy-free, low-calorie option that provides healthy fats and minerals.

- Honey (if used) can provide a natural sweetener and additional antioxidants.

The combination of these ingredients creates a delicious and nutritious smoothie that can be enjoyed as a healthy snack or meal replacement. It's a great way to incorporate more plant-based foods into your diet and support overall health and well-being as you age.

How would you rate this dish?

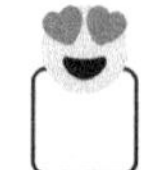 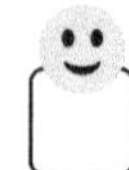 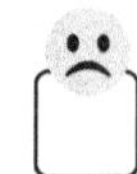 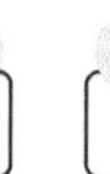 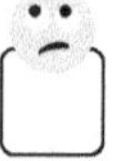 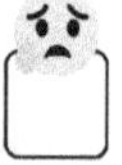

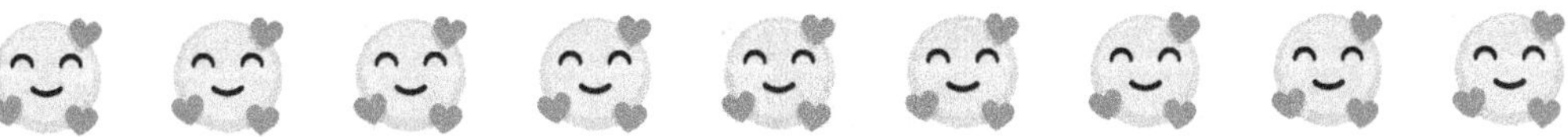

113. Freshly squeezed orange juice

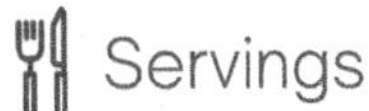 Prep Time :   Cook Time :   Servings :

Is this dish easy or difficult for you to make?

 ◯   ◯

Write 5 ....
friends
with ....
whom
you ....
want to
share ....
this
dish ....

INGREDIENTS

- 4-5 medium oranges, washed

---

1. Cut the oranges in half crosswise.

2. Using a citrus juicer or reamer, squeeze the juice from each orange half into a pitcher or container.

3. Stir the juice to combine.

4. Serve the freshly squeezed orange juice immediately, or refrigerate until ready to serve.

This recipe supports the MIND diet for seniors over 60 because:

- Oranges are a fruit, which are a key component of the MIND diet's emphasis on plant-based foods.

- Freshly squeezed orange juice is a natural, unprocessed beverage that is free of added sugars or other additives.

- Oranges are a good source of vitamin C, which is an important nutrient for overall health and cognitive function.

The MIND diet has been shown to help reduce the risk of cognitive decline and Alzheimer's disease in older adults. Enjoying a glass of freshly squeezed orange juice can be a refreshing and nutritious part of a MIND diet-friendly meal plan.

Some tips for making the best freshly squeezed orange juice:

- Use ripe, juicy oranges for maximum flavor and sweetness.
- Roll the oranges on the counter before cutting to help release more juice.
- Strain the juice through a fine-mesh sieve to remove any pulp or seeds, if desired.
- Serve the juice chilled or over ice for a refreshing treat.

How would you rate this dish?

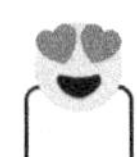 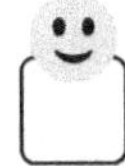  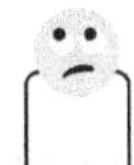 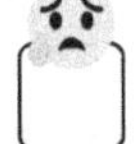

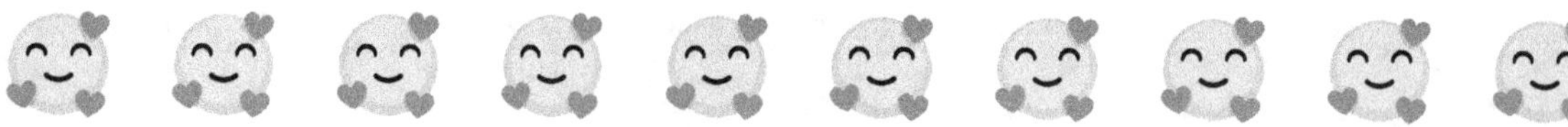

114. Herbal tea with lemon

Prep Time : 

Cook Time :

Servings :

Is this dish easy or difficult for you to make?

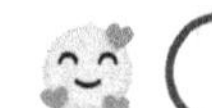 ◯   ◯

Write 5 friends with whom you want to share this dish

....

....

....

....

....

INGREDIENTS

- 1 herbal tea bag (such as chamomile, peppermint, or ginger)
- 1 cup boiling water
- 1 slice of lemon

1. Bring 1 cup of water to a boil in a small saucepan or kettle.

2. Place the herbal tea bag in a mug or teacup.

3. Pour the boiling water over the tea bag.

4. Allow the tea to steep for 5-7 minutes, or according to the package instructions.

5. Remove the tea bag and stir in a slice of fresh lemon.

6. Enjoy the herbal tea hot or let it cool slightly before drinking.

This simple herbal tea with lemon is a great option for seniors over 60 for a few reasons:

1. Herbal teas are caffeine-free, which can be beneficial for older adults who may be more sensitive to the effects of caffeine.

2. Certain herbal teas, like chamomile and peppermint, have been shown to have calming and soothing properties that can help promote relaxation and better sleep.

3. Lemon provides a refreshing and tart flavor, as well as a boost of vitamin C, which is important for immune function and overall health.

4. Staying hydrated is crucial for seniors, and sipping on a warm, comforting beverage like this herbal tea can help encourage fluid intake.

Overall, this herbal tea with lemon is a simple, healthy, and delicious option that can support the well-being of seniors over 60. Enjoy it as a relaxing afternoon or evening treat.

How would you rate this dish?

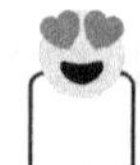 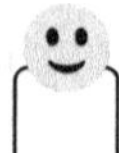  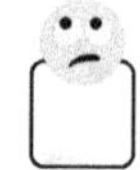 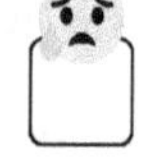

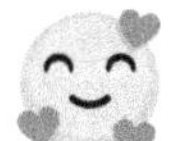 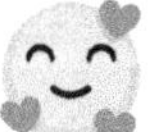 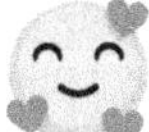 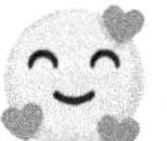 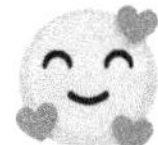 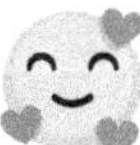 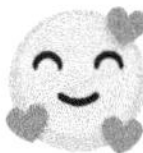 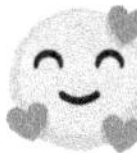 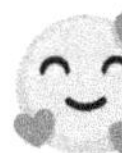 

115. Matcha green tea

Prep Time :   **Cook Time :**   **Servings :**

Is this dish easy or difficult for you to make?

 ◯   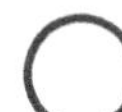 ◯

Write 5 friends with whom you want to share this dish

....
....
....
....
....

INGREDIENTS

- 1 teaspoon high-quality matcha green tea powder
- 2-3 ounces hot water (around 175°F/80°C)
- Optional: 1-2 teaspoons honey or maple syrup (to sweeten)

1. Gather your matcha tea bowl, a small whisk (called a chasen), and a spoon.

2. Sift the matcha powder into the bowl using a fine-mesh sieve. This helps break up any clumps.

3. Add 2-3 ounces of hot water (not boiling) to the bowl.

4. Using the whisk, briskly whisk the matcha and water together in a zig-zag motion until the tea is frothy and smooth, about 30 seconds to 1 minute.

5. If desired, stir in 1-2 teaspoons of honey or maple syrup to sweeten the tea.

6. Enjoy the matcha tea immediately while it's hot and frothy.

Matcha green tea is an excellent beverage choice for seniors over 60 for several reasons:

- Matcha is packed with antioxidants, vitamins, and minerals that can support overall health and well-being.

- The L-theanine in matcha can help promote calm focus and relaxation without the jitteriness of coffee.

- Matcha may help boost metabolism and support healthy weight management.

- The ritual of preparing and drinking matcha can be a soothing, mindful experience.

When selecting matcha, be sure to choose a high-quality, ceremonial-grade powder for the best flavor and health benefits. Enjoy your matcha tea hot or over ice for a refreshing and nourishing beverage.

How would you rate this dish?

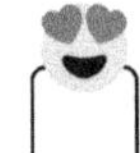 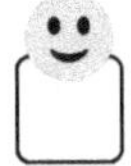  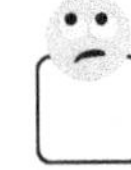 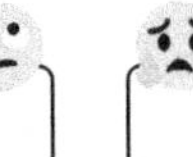

www.ingramcontent.com/pod-product-compliance
Lightning Source LLC
Chambersburg PA
CBHW081550250726
48653CB00009B/3363

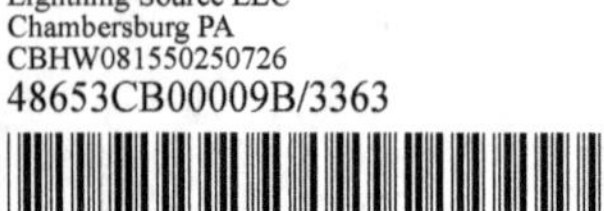